ESSENTIAL RHEUMATOLOGY

Case Scenarios for Effective Diagnosis and Management

Essam Abdelhakim

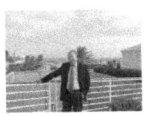

Copyright © 2024 Essam abdelhakim

All rights reserved

The characters and events portrayed in this book are fictitious. Any similarity to real persons, living or dead, is coincidental and not intended by the author.

No part of this book may be reproduced, or stored in a retrieval system, or transmitted in any form or by any means, electronic, mechanical, photocopying, recording, or otherwise, without express written permission of the publisher.

Cover design by: Art Painter
Library of Congress Control Number: 2018675309
Printed in the United States of America

CONTENTS

Title Page
Copyright
Introduction
Case 1: Rheumatoid Arthritis   1
Case 2: Systemic Lupus Erythematosus (SLE)   4
Case 3: Gout   7
Case 4: Ankylosing Spondylitis   9
Case 5: Polymyalgia Rheumatica   11
Case 6: Sjögren's Syndrome   13
Case 7: Psoriatic Arthritis   15
Case 8: Fibromyalgia   17
Case 9: Giant Cell Arteritis (GCA)   19
Case 10: Scleroderma   21
Case 11: Reactive Arthritis   24
Case 12: Osteoarthritis   26
Case 13: Behçet's Disease   28
Case 14: Gout(2)   30
Case 15: Methotrexate in Rheumatoid Arthritis   32
Case 16: Hydroxychloroquine in Systemic Lupus Erythematosus (SLE)   35
Case 17: Leflunomide in Psoriatic Arthritis   38

Case 18: Tumor Necrosis Factor (TNF) Inhibitors in Ankylosing Spondylitis — 40

Case 19: Rheumatoid Arthritis Prognosis — 43

Case 20: Systemic Lupus Erythematosus (SLE) Follow-Up — 46

Case 21: Ankylosing Spondylitis Prognosis — 49

Case 22: Gout Follow-Up — 52

Case 23: Diagnosing Rheumatoid Arthritis(2) — 54

Case 24: Evaluating Systemic Lupus Erythematosus (SLE) — 56

Case 25: Investigating Gout — 58

Case 26: Investigating Psoriatic Arthritis — 60

Case 27: Evaluating Ankylosing Spondylitis — 62

Case 28: Investigating Sjögren's Syndrome — 64

Case 29: Investigating Osteoarthritis — 66

Case 30: Investigating Dermatomyositis — 68

Case 31: Investigating Scleroderma — 70

Case 32: Investigating Mixed Connective Tissue Disease (MCTD) — 72

Case 33: Limited Systemic Sclerosis — 74

Case 34: Large Vessel Vasculitis — 76

Case 35: Diffuse Systemic Sclerosis — 78

Case 36: Regional Pain Syndromes — 80

Case 37: Kawasaki Disease — 82

Case 38: Managing Complications of Systemic Sclerosis — 84

Case 39: Myofascial Pain Syndrome — 86

Case 40: Paget's Disease — 88

Case 41: Soft Tissue Rheumatism — 90

Case 42: Long-Term Management of Systemic Sclerosis — 92

Case 43: Polymyositis — 94

Case 44: Dermatomyositis(2) — 96

Case 45: Medium Vessel Vasculitis	98
Case 46: Small Vessel Vasculitis	100
Case 47: Fibromyalgia(2)	102
Case 48: Juvenile Idiopathic Arthritis (JIA)	104
Case 49: Systemic Juvenile Idiopathic Arthritis (sJIA)	106
Case 50: Other Pediatric Rheumatic Conditions	108
Case 51: Pregnancy and Rheumatic Diseases	110
Case 52: Geriatric Rheumatology Considerations	112
Case 53: Pregnancy with Rheumatic Disease	114
Case 54: Geriatric Patient with Gout	116
Case 55: Septic Arthritis	118
Case 56: Catastrophic Antiphospholipid Syndrome	120
Case 57: Acute Gout Attack with Infection	122
Case 58: Pulmonary Vasculitis Emergency	124
Case 59: Adult Still's Disease	126
Case 60: Mixed Connective Tissue Disease (MCTD)	128
Case 61: Eosinophilic Granulomatosis with Polyangiitis (EGPA)	130
Case 62: DMARDs in Rheumatoid Arthritis	132
Case 63: Biologics in Psoriatic Arthritis	134
Case 64: Novel Therapies in SLE	136
Case 65: Managing Treatment-Related Complications	138
Case 66: Collaborative Care for a Patient with Osteoarthritis	140
Case 67: Rheumatoid Arthritis and Orthopedic Management	142
Case 68: Fibromyalgia and Multidisciplinary Approach	144
Case 69: Interdisciplinary Approach in Gout Management	146
Case 70: Mechanical Low Back Pain	148

Case 71: Inflammatory Low Back Pain — 150
Case 72: Differential Diagnosis Approach — 152
Case 73: Chronic Low Back Pain Management — 154
Case 74: Monoarthritis — 156
Case 75: Oligoarthritis — 158
Case 76: Polyarthritis — 160
Case 77: Systemic Symptoms in Rheumatic Disease — 162
About The Author — 165
Disclosure — 167

INTRODUCTION

In "Rheumatology Case Scenarios," we present an invaluable resource for medical professionals navigating the complexities of rheumatologic disorders.

Each chapter is structured to facilitate learning through a systematic approach:

Clinical Scenarios(77 Cases): Each case presents a patient with specific symptoms and clinical findings, allowing readers to engage with real-life situations that challenge their diagnostic abilities.

Multiple-Choice Questions (MCQs): Accompanying each scenario, a set of MCQs tests the readers understanding and application of knowledge in diagnosing and managing rheumatic conditions.

Answers and Explanations: Detailed explanations follow the MCQs, clarifying the rationale behind the correct answers and providing insights into common pitfalls in diagnosis and treatment.

Tips and Pearls: Practical tips and clinical pearls are offered to enhance patient care, emphasizing key aspects of rheumatology practice that can improve outcomes and guide treatment decisions.

Pitfalls to Avoid: Each scenario concludes with a discussion of potential pitfalls, helping medical professionals recognize and sidestep common errors in managing rheumatic diseases.

CASE 1: RHEUMATOID ARTHRITIS

Clinical Scenario:
A 45-year-old woman presents to the clinic with complaints of joint pain and stiffness in both hands for the past 6 months. The pain is worse in the morning and lasts for about 1 hour before easing.

On examination, there is swelling and tenderness in the metacarpophalangeal and proximal interphalangeal joints bilaterally. She also reports fatigue and mild fever. Her ESR and CRP are elevated. Rheumatoid factor (RF) and anti-cyclic citrullinated peptide (anti-CCP) antibodies are positive.

1. What is the most likely diagnosis for this patient?
   A. Osteoarthritis
   B. Rheumatoid Arthritis
   C. Systemic Lupus Erythematosus
   D. Psoriatic Arthritis
2. Which of the following is the most appropriate initial treatment?
   A. Methotrexate
   B. NSAIDs
   C. Corticosteroids
   D. Hydroxychloroquine
3. What is a typical radiographic finding in rheumatoid arthritis?
   A. Joint space narrowing and erosions

B. Osteophyte formation
   C. Syndesmophytes
   D. Bone sclerosis

Answers:
1. **B. Rheumatoid Arthritis**
2. **A. Methotrexate**
3. **A. Joint space narrowing and erosions**

Explanation:

- **Diagnosis:** Rheumatoid arthritis (RA) is an autoimmune condition characterized by chronic synovial inflammation leading to joint damage. The clinical presentation of symmetric joint involvement, morning stiffness, and positive RF and anti-CCP antibodies strongly support this diagnosis.
- **Initial Treatment:** Methotrexate is the first-line disease-modifying antirheumatic drug (DMARD) for RA. NSAIDs and corticosteroids can be used for symptomatic relief, but DMARDs are required to prevent disease progression.
- **Radiographic Findings:** Erosions and joint space narrowing on X-ray are classic findings in RA due to chronic inflammation and cartilage destruction.

Tips & Pearls:

- Always assess for both RF and anti-CCP antibodies when suspecting RA. Anti-CCP is more specific and indicates a higher risk of joint damage.
- Start DMARDs early to prevent irreversible joint damage and long-term disability.
- Monitor for methotrexate toxicity, including liver function and pulmonary toxicity.

Pitfalls to Avoid:
- Delaying DMARD therapy in the early stages of rheumatoid arthritis can lead to severe joint deformities.
- Avoid diagnosing RA based on RF alone, as it can be positive in other conditions like Sjögren's syndrome or even healthy individuals.
- Underestimating the importance of regular monitoring for side effects of methotrexate and other DMARDs can lead to complications.

CASE 2: SYSTEMIC LUPUS ERYTHEMATOSUS (SLE)

Clinical Scenario:

A 25-year-old woman presents with fatigue, joint pain, and a rash on her cheeks for 3 months. She has noticed hair thinning and has experienced intermittent fevers.

Physical examination reveals a malar rash and mild swelling of her wrists. Blood tests show positive ANA, anti-dsDNA antibodies, and low C3/C4 levels.

1. What is the most likely diagnosis?
   A. Rheumatoid Arthritis
   B. Systemic Lupus Erythematosus
   C. Sjögren's Syndrome
   D. Dermatomyositis

2. Which of the following would be an appropriate treatment for this patient?
   A. Methotrexate
   B. Hydroxychloroquine
   C. NSAIDs alone
   D. Prednisone

3. What is the most specific antibody for diagnosing SLE?

A. ANA
B. Anti-dsDNA
C. Anti-RNP
D. Anti-SSA

Answers:
1. **B. Systemic Lupus Erythematosus**
2. **B. Hydroxychloroquine**
3. **B. Anti-dsDNA**

Explanation:
- **Diagnosis:** SLE is an autoimmune disorder commonly affecting young women. The presence of a malar rash, positive ANA, and anti-dsDNA antibodies confirms the diagnosis.
- **Treatment:** Hydroxychloroquine is the cornerstone of SLE treatment. It helps manage symptoms and prevents flares. NSAIDs and corticosteroids can be used for symptomatic relief.
- **Antibody Testing:** Anti-dsDNA antibodies are highly specific for SLE, particularly in the context of renal involvement.

Tips & Pearls:
- Always check complement levels (C3, C4) as they are often low during active disease.
- Hydroxychloroquine is well tolerated and should be continued long-term in most SLE patients.
- Regular eye exams are necessary while on hydroxychloroquine due to the risk of retinopathy.

Pitfalls to Avoid:
- Don't rely solely on ANA for diagnosis, as it is non-specific and can be positive in many conditions.
- Avoid high doses of corticosteroids long term due to

the risk of severe side effects.

CASE 3: GOUT

Clinical Scenario:

A 68-year-old man presents with severe pain in his right big toe. The pain began suddenly last night and is associated with redness and swelling.

He reports a history of hypertension and is on diuretics. On examination, the first metatarsophalangeal joint is erythematous, swollen, and tender to touch. Serum uric acid is elevated.

1. What is the most likely diagnosis?
    A. Septic arthritis
    B. Gout
    C. Pseudogout
    D. Osteoarthritis
2. Which medication is most appropriate for acute treatment?
    A. Allopurinol
    B. Colchicine
    C. Methotrexate
    D. Hydroxychloroquine
3. What would be the expected finding on joint aspiration?
    A. Positively birefringent crystals
    B. Negatively birefringent crystals
    C. Gram-positive cocci
    D. Calcium pyrophosphate crystals

Answers:

1. **B. Gout**

2. **B. Colchicine**
3. **B. Negatively birefringent crystals**

Explanation:

- **Diagnosis:** Gout presents with acute monoarthritis, often affecting the first MTP joint (podagra). Diuretics and hyperuricemia increase the risk.
- **Treatment:** Colchicine is used for acute attacks, while allopurinol is for long-term urate-lowering therapy.
- **Joint Aspiration:** Gout is characterized by needle-shaped, negatively birefringent urate crystals under polarized light microscopy.

Tips & Pearls:

- Uric acid-lowering therapy like allopurinol should be initiated only after the acute attack has subsided.
- Diuretics can increase uric acid levels, so consider alternatives in patients with recurrent gout.
- Colchicine should be dosed cautiously to avoid gastrointestinal side effects.

Pitfalls to Avoid:

- Avoid starting or stopping allopurinol during an acute gout flare as it may worsen the attack.
- Missing septic arthritis, which can present similarly, is a dangerous pitfall.

CASE 4: ANKYLOSING SPONDYLITIS

Clinical Scenario:

A 30-year-old man presents with chronic lower back pain and stiffness, particularly in the morning, which improves with activity.

He also reports occasional eye pain and redness. Examination reveals limited lumbar spine mobility and tenderness over the sacroiliac joints. HLA-B27 is positive.

1. What is the most likely diagnosis?
   A. Rheumatoid Arthritis
   B. Ankylosing Spondylitis
   C. Psoriatic Arthritis
   D. Fibromyalgia
2. What is the hallmark radiographic finding?
   A. Bamboo spine
   B. Osteophytes
   C. Joint space narrowing
   D. Erosions
3. What is the first-line treatment for this condition?
   A. NSAIDs
   B. Methotrexate
   C. Corticosteroids
   D. Hydroxychloroquine

Answers:

1. **B. Ankylosing Spondylitis**

2. **A. Bamboo spine**
3. **A. NSAIDs**

Explanation:

- **Diagnosis:** Ankylosing spondylitis is a chronic inflammatory disease affecting the spine and sacroiliac joints, often associated with HLA-B27 positivity.
- **Radiographic Findings:** Bamboo spine, due to vertebral body fusion, is characteristic.
- **Treatment:** NSAIDs are the first-line treatment to reduce inflammation and pain.

Tips & Pearls:

- Encourage regular physical therapy to maintain spine mobility.
- Monitor for extra-articular manifestations, including uveitis and inflammatory bowel disease.
- Anti-TNF agents are recommended for those not responding to NSAIDs.

Pitfalls to Avoid:

- Misdiagnosing mechanical back pain or fibromyalgia in patients with inflammatory back pain.
- Neglecting extra-articular manifestations, especially uveitis.

CASE 5: POLYMYALGIA RHEUMATICA

Clinical Scenario:

A 72-year-old woman presents with stiffness and pain in her shoulders and hips, particularly in the morning. The symptoms have gradually worsened over the past 3 months.

She denies muscle weakness. On examination, she has tenderness in the shoulders and hips but full range of motion. Her ESR is elevated at 60 mm/hr.

1. What is the most likely diagnosis?
   A. Rheumatoid Arthritis
   B. Polymyalgia Rheumatica
   C. Osteoarthritis
   D. Fibromyalgia
2. What is the treatment of choice?
   A. Methotrexate
   B. NSAIDs
   C. Low-dose corticosteroids
   D. Hydroxychloroquine
3. Which condition is often associated with this diagnosis?
   A. Systemic Lupus Erythematosus
   B. Giant Cell Arteritis
   C. Scleroderma
   D. Ankylosing Spondylitis

Answers:

1. **B. Polymyalgia Rheumatica**
2. **C. Low-dose corticosteroids**
3. **B. Giant Cell Arteritis**

Explanation:

- **Diagnosis:** Polymyalgia rheumatica (PMR) presents with proximal stiffness and pain without muscle weakness in elderly patients. An elevated ESR supports the diagnosis.
- **Treatment:** Low-dose corticosteroids (10-20 mg of prednisone) typically lead to rapid improvement.
- **Association:** PMR is closely linked with giant cell arteritis (GCA), and patients should be monitored for symptoms like headache and visual disturbances.

Tips & Pearls:

- A rapid response to low-dose steroids strongly supports the diagnosis of PMR.
- Be vigilant for symptoms of GCA, such as jaw claudication and visual loss.
- Relapses may occur, requiring longer corticosteroid tapering.

Pitfalls to Avoid:

- Misdiagnosing PMR as fibromyalgia or osteoarthritis can delay appropriate treatment.
- Failure to recognize GCA in PMR patients can lead to serious complications, including blindness.

CASE 6: SJÖGREN'S SYNDROME

Clinical Scenario:

A 50-year-old woman presents with dry eyes and dry mouth for the past year. She has difficulty swallowing dry food and constantly uses artificial tears.

She has a history of rheumatoid arthritis. Examination reveals dry oral mucosa and a reduced tear film on Schirmer's test. ANA and anti-SSA antibodies are positive.

1. What is the most likely diagnosis?
    A. Rheumatoid Arthritis
    B. Systemic Lupus Erythematosus
    C. Sjögren's Syndrome
    D. Scleroderma

2. What is the most appropriate management for this patient?
    A. Methotrexate
    B. Hydroxychloroquine
    C. Pilocarpine
    D. NSAIDs

3. What complication is most commonly associated with Sjögren's syndrome?
    A. Lymphoma
    B. Interstitial lung disease
    C. Renal failure
    D. Coronary artery disease

Answers:

1. **C. Sjögren's Syndrome**
2. **C. Pilocarpine**
3. **A. Lymphoma**

Explanation:

- **Diagnosis:** Sjögren's syndrome is an autoimmune condition characterized by dry eyes and dry mouth. Positive anti-SSA antibodies help confirm the diagnosis.
- **Treatment:** Pilocarpine, a cholinergic agent, helps stimulate saliva and tear production.
- **Complication:** Patients with Sjögren's syndrome have an increased risk of developing non-Hodgkin lymphoma.

Tips & Pearls:

- Consider salivary gland biopsy for diagnosis in cases of diagnostic uncertainty.
- Artificial tears and saliva substitutes provide symptomatic relief for dry eyes and mouth.
- Monitor for lymphoma development, especially in cases of persistent glandular swelling.

Pitfalls to Avoid:

- Overlooking the risk of lymphoma in patients with Sjögren's syndrome.
- Failing to address dental care, as dry mouth predisposes to dental caries.

CASE 7: PSORIATIC ARTHRITIS

Clinical Scenario:

A 35-year-old man presents with pain and swelling in his fingers and toes. He also has a history of psoriasis with patches on his scalp and elbows.

Examination reveals dactylitis ("sausage digits") in the second and third fingers and pitting of the nails. His X-ray shows erosion and "pencil-in-cup" deformities of the distal interphalangeal joints.

1. What is the most likely diagnosis?
   A. Rheumatoid Arthritis
   B. Osteoarthritis
   C. Psoriatic Arthritis
   D. Reactive Arthritis

2. Which of the following is commonly associated with this condition?
   A. Uveitis
   B. Renal failure
   C. Liver cirrhosis
   D. Myocarditis

3. What is the first-line treatment for this condition?
   A. NSAIDs
   B. Methotrexate
   C. Anti-TNF agents
   D. Hydroxychloroquine

Answers:
1. **C. Psoriatic Arthritis**
2. **A. Uveitis**
3. **B. Methotrexate**

Explanation:
- **Diagnosis:** Psoriatic arthritis (PsA) is characterized by dactylitis, nail pitting, and joint deformities. It often affects patients with a history of psoriasis.
- **Association:** PsA is linked with uveitis, which may present as eye pain and redness.
- **Treatment:** Methotrexate is a common first-line therapy, with anti-TNF agents used in severe cases.

Tips & Pearls:
- Early recognition of PsA is key to preventing joint damage.
- Check for skin and nail involvement in all patients with inflammatory arthritis.
- Biologic agents are effective for patients who fail to respond to DMARDs like methotrexate.

Pitfalls to Avoid:
- Failing to screen for PsA in patients with psoriasis can delay diagnosis.
- Avoid underestimating the risk of ocular complications, such as uveitis.

CASE 8: FIBROMYALGIA

Clinical Scenario:

A 28-year-old woman presents with widespread musculoskeletal pain for the past 6 months.

She reports feeling fatigued, having difficulty sleeping, and experiencing "brain fog."

Physical examination reveals tenderness at multiple soft tissue points but no joint swelling or inflammation. Lab results are normal, including ESR, CRP, and ANA.

1. What is the most likely diagnosis?
    A. Rheumatoid Arthritis
    B. Polymyalgia Rheumatica
    C. Fibromyalgia
    D. Systemic Lupus Erythematosus
2. Which of the following is the cornerstone of treatment?
    A. Corticosteroids
    B. Methotrexate
    C. Physical therapy and exercise
    D. NSAIDs
3. What medication is commonly used for symptom management in fibromyalgia?
    A. Prednisone
    B. Duloxetine
    C. Hydroxychloroquine

D. Colchicine

Answers:

1. **C. Fibromyalgia**
2. **C. Physical therapy and exercise**
3. **B. Duloxetine**

Explanation:

- **Diagnosis:** Fibromyalgia is a chronic pain syndrome characterized by widespread pain, fatigue, and cognitive issues without inflammatory findings.
- **Treatment:** Exercise and cognitive behavioral therapy are key in managing symptoms.
- **Medication:** Duloxetine and other serotonin-norepinephrine reuptake inhibitors (SNRIs) are often used for pain relief.

Tips & Pearls:

- Encourage patients to adopt a multidisciplinary approach, including exercise, sleep hygiene, and counseling.
- Address the psychological aspects of fibromyalgia, as anxiety and depression often coexist.
- Use medications like duloxetine or pregabalin for symptomatic relief.

Pitfalls to Avoid:

- Misdiagnosing fibromyalgia as an inflammatory arthritis or autoimmune disease.
- Over-relying on medications without encouraging lifestyle modifications and physical therapy.

CASE 9: GIANT CELL ARTERITIS (GCA)

Clinical Scenario:

A 75-year-old woman presents with a new-onset headache, jaw pain while chewing, and visual disturbances. She also complains of scalp tenderness when combing her hair.

Physical examination reveals tenderness over the temporal arteries. Her ESR is elevated at 85 mm/hr.

1. What is the most likely diagnosis?
    A. Polymyalgia Rheumatica
    B. Giant Cell Arteritis
    C. Temporal Lobe Epilepsy
    D. Migraine
2. What is the best initial treatment?
    A. Methotrexate
    B. NSAIDs
    C. High-dose corticosteroids
    D. Aspirin
3. What is the most feared complication of this condition?
    A. Stroke
    B. Vision loss
    C. Jaw dislocation
    D. Scalp necrosis

Answers:

1. **B. Giant Cell Arteritis**

2. **C. High-dose corticosteroids**
3. **B. Vision loss**

Explanation:

- **Diagnosis:** GCA (also known as temporal arteritis) commonly presents with headache, jaw claudication, and visual symptoms in elderly individuals. An elevated ESR supports the diagnosis.
- **Treatment:** Immediate initiation of high-dose corticosteroids is crucial to prevent vision loss.
- **Complication:** Vision loss due to ischemic optic neuropathy is the most feared complication of GCA.

Tips & Pearls:

- Biopsy of the temporal artery is the gold standard for diagnosis, but treatment should not be delayed while waiting for biopsy results.
- Regular follow-up is required to taper corticosteroids and monitor for side effects like osteoporosis.
- GCA is closely linked with polymyalgia rheumatica, and both conditions may coexist.

Pitfalls to Avoid:

- Delaying treatment while waiting for biopsy results can lead to irreversible vision loss.
- Misdiagnosing GCA as a migraine or tension headache may delay appropriate treatment.

CASE 10: SCLERODERMA

Clinical Scenario:

A 45-year-old woman presents with tightness of the skin on her hands and face, along with difficulty swallowing.

She reports Raynaud's phenomenon and has noticed her fingers turning white and blue in cold weather.

On examination, her skin appears thickened and shiny over her hands. ANA is positive, and anti-centromere antibodies are present.

1. What is the most likely diagnosis?
   A. Rheumatoid Arthritis
   B. Scleroderma
   C. Systemic Lupus Erythematosus
   D. Sjögren's Syndrome

2. What is the most specific autoantibody for limited cutaneous scleroderma?
   A. Anti-dsDNA
   B. Anti-SSA
   C. Anti-centromere
   D. Anti-Scl-70

3. Which of the following is a common complication of scleroderma?
   A. Renal crisis
   B. Pulmonary fibrosis

C. Pericarditis
D. Hepatitis

Answers:
1. **B. Scleroderma**
2. **C. Anti-centromere**
3. **B. Pulmonary fibrosis**

Explanation:
- **Diagnosis:** Scleroderma is characterized by skin thickening, Raynaud's phenomenon, and systemic involvement. The presence of anti-centromere antibodies suggests the limited cutaneous form.
- **Antibody Testing:** Anti-centromere antibodies are associated with limited scleroderma, while anti-Scl-70 is linked with the diffuse form.
- **Complications:** Pulmonary fibrosis is a common and serious complication of scleroderma, particularly in the diffuse form.

Tips & Pearls:
- Raynaud's phenomenon is often the first symptom of scleroderma and should prompt further investigation.
- Early recognition of pulmonary involvement is crucial to manage interstitial lung disease.
- Calcium channel blockers can help manage Raynaud's phenomenon.

Pitfalls to Avoid:
- Failing to recognize scleroderma in patients presenting with Raynaud's phenomenon may delay diagnosis and treatment.
- Overlooking pulmonary involvement can lead to significant morbidity in patients with diffuse

scleroderma.

CASE 11: REACTIVE ARTHRITIS

Clinical Scenario:

A 30-year-old man presents with joint pain in his knees and ankles, along with redness of the eyes and dysuria. He reports a recent history of diarrhea a week ago.

On examination, he has conjunctivitis, swollen and tender knee joints, and a scaly rash on the soles of his feet.

1. What is the most likely diagnosis?
   A. Psoriatic Arthritis
   B. Reactive Arthritis
   C. Rheumatoid Arthritis
   D. Ankylosing Spondylitis

2. Which of the following infections is commonly associated with this condition?
   A. Staphylococcus aureus
   B. Streptococcus pyogenes
   C. Chlamydia trachomatis
   D. Mycobacterium tuberculosis

3. What is the appropriate initial treatment?
   A. NSAIDs
   B. Methotrexate
   C. Corticosteroids
   D. Colchicine

Answers:

1. **B. Reactive Arthritis**
2. **C. Chlamydia trachomatis**
3. **A. NSAIDs**

Explanation:
- **Diagnosis:** Reactive arthritis is a seronegative spondyloarthropathy that presents with arthritis, conjunctivitis, and urethritis following an infection (classically gastrointestinal or genitourinary).
- **Infection:** Chlamydia trachomatis is a common trigger for reactive arthritis, although gastrointestinal infections (e.g., Salmonella, Shigella) can also be implicated.
- **Treatment:** NSAIDs are the first-line treatment for reactive arthritis, providing relief from pain and inflammation.

Tips & Pearls:
- The classic triad of arthritis, urethritis, and conjunctivitis is characteristic of reactive arthritis.
- Reactive arthritis typically occurs 1-4 weeks after an infection.
- Consider screening for sexually transmitted infections in cases of reactive arthritis.

Pitfalls to Avoid:
- Missing the diagnosis in patients with a history of recent infection and arthritis.
- Overlooking the possibility of a sexually transmitted infection as a trigger.

CASE 12: OSTEOARTHRITIS

Clinical Scenario:

A 65-year-old man presents with joint pain in his knees, particularly after long walks. He reports stiffness that lasts for a few minutes in the morning and pain that worsens throughout the day.

On examination, there is crepitus in both knees and bony enlargements of the distal interphalangeal joints.

1. What is the most likely diagnosis?
    A. Rheumatoid Arthritis
    B. Osteoarthritis
    C. Gout
    D. Pseudogout
2. What radiographic findings are typical of this condition?
    A. Erosions
    B. Osteophytes
    C. Joint subluxation
    D. Joint space widening
3. What is the first-line pharmacological treatment for osteoarthritis?
    A. Corticosteroids
    B. Methotrexate
    C. NSAIDs
    D. Hydroxychloroquine

Answers:
1. **B. Osteoarthritis**
2. **B. Osteophytes**
3. **C. NSAIDs**

Explanation:
- **Diagnosis:** Osteoarthritis is a degenerative joint disease commonly affecting weight-bearing joints like the knees. The presence of bony enlargements and joint crepitus is typical.
- **Radiographic Findings:** Osteophytes, joint space narrowing, and subchondral sclerosis are classic findings.
- **Treatment:** NSAIDs are the first-line treatment for pain relief in osteoarthritis.

Tips & Pearls:
- Weight loss and physical therapy are important non-pharmacological treatments.
- Consider intra-articular corticosteroids for patients with severe pain not responding to NSAIDs.
- Encourage low-impact exercises like swimming or cycling to maintain joint mobility.

Pitfalls to Avoid:
- Over-relying on medications without incorporating lifestyle changes such as weight management and exercise.
- Failing to distinguish between osteoarthritis and inflammatory arthritis (e.g., rheumatoid arthritis).

CASE 13: BEHÇET'S DISEASE

Clinical Scenario:

A 40-year-old man presents with recurrent painful oral ulcers, genital ulcers, and red, tender bumps on his lower legs.

He also reports episodes of eye pain and redness. Examination reveals multiple aphthous ulcers in the oral mucosa and erythema nodosum on the legs. He is of Mediterranean descent.

1. What is the most likely diagnosis?
   A. Systemic Lupus Erythematosus
   B. Behçet's Disease
   C. Reactive Arthritis
   D. Sjögren's Syndrome
2. What is the most appropriate initial treatment for this condition?
   A. Methotrexate
   B. NSAIDs
   C. Corticosteroids
   D. Hydroxychloroquine
3. Which of the following complications is associated with Behçet's disease?
   A. Pulmonary embolism
   B. Aortic dissection
   C. Uveitis
   D. Cardiomyopathy

Answers:
1. **B. Behçet's Disease**
2. **C. Corticosteroids**
3. **C. Uveitis**

Explanation:
- **Diagnosis:** Behçet's disease is characterized by recurrent oral and genital ulcers, erythema nodosum, and uveitis. It is more common in individuals of Mediterranean or Middle Eastern descent.
- **Treatment:** Corticosteroids are commonly used to control acute flares, especially for skin and mucosal involvement.
- **Complication:** Uveitis is a frequent and potentially serious complication of Behçet's disease, requiring prompt ophthalmologic evaluation.

Tips & Pearls:
- Behçet's disease should be considered in patients with recurrent oral and genital ulcers and eye involvement.
- Immunosuppressive therapies may be required for severe or organ-threatening manifestations.
- HLA-B51 is associated with an increased risk of Behçet's disease.

Pitfalls to Avoid:
- Misdiagnosing Behçet's disease as simple aphthous stomatitis or herpes simplex virus infection.
- Failing to recognize ocular involvement can lead to vision loss.

CASE 14: GOUT(2)

Clinical Scenario:

A 50-year-old man presents with sudden onset of severe pain, redness, and swelling in his right big toe. He has a history of hypertension and is taking thiazide diuretics. He admits to drinking alcohol regularly.

On examination, his first metatarsophalangeal joint is warm, erythematous, and tender. Joint aspiration reveals needle-shaped crystals under polarized light.

1. What is the most likely diagnosis?
   A. Rheumatoid Arthritis
   B. Septic Arthritis
   C. Gout
   D. Pseudogout

2. Which of the following is the most common risk factor for this condition?
   A. Alcohol consumption
   B. Diabetes mellitus
   C. Hypothyroidism
   D. Hypertension

3. What is the treatment of choice for acute gout flares?
   A. NSAIDs
   B. Colchicine
   C. Corticosteroids
   D. Allopurinol

Answers:

1. **C. Gout**

2. **A. Alcohol consumption**
3. **A. NSAIDs**

Explanation:
- **Diagnosis:** Gout is characterized by the deposition of monosodium urate crystals in joints, leading to acute inflammation. The first metatarsophalangeal joint is commonly affected.
- **Risk Factors:** Alcohol consumption and the use of thiazide diuretics are common triggers for gout flares.
- **Treatment:** NSAIDs are the first-line treatment for managing acute gout attacks.

Tips & Pearls:
- Uric acid levels may be normal during an acute gout flare, so diagnosis is best confirmed by joint aspiration.
- Dietary modifications, including reducing alcohol and purine intake, can help prevent future gout attacks.
- Chronic gout may require urate-lowering therapy such as allopurinol.

Pitfalls to Avoid:
- Treating gout flares with urate-lowering therapy during an acute episode may worsen symptoms.
- Misdiagnosing gout as septic arthritis can lead to unnecessary antibiotic use.

CASE 15: METHOTREXATE IN RHEUMATOID ARTHRITIS

Clinical Scenario:

A 45-year-old woman with newly diagnosed rheumatoid arthritis is started on methotrexate. She is advised to take it once weekly, along with folic acid supplementation.

Two months later, she returns to the clinic complaining of fatigue, mouth sores, and occasional nausea. Laboratory tests show a slight increase in liver enzymes.

1. What is the most likely cause of this patient's symptoms?
    A. Methotrexate toxicity
    B. Rheumatoid arthritis flare
    C. Folic acid deficiency
    D. NSAID-related side effects
2. What is the most appropriate next step in managing this patient?
    A. Increase methotrexate dose
    B. Stop methotrexate and switch to biologics
    C. Add folic acid or increase the dose
    D. Start corticosteroids

3. Which of the following is a common side effect of methotrexate?
   A. Nephrotoxicity
   B. Hepatotoxicity
   C. Retinopathy
   D. Pulmonary fibrosis

Answers:
1. **A. Methotrexate toxicity**
2. **C. Add folic acid or increase the dose**
3. **B. Hepatotoxicity**

Explanation:
- **Diagnosis:** Methotrexate can cause side effects like mouth sores and fatigue, which can be alleviated by folic acid supplementation.
- **Management:** Increasing folic acid supplementation is a common strategy to reduce methotrexate side effects. Liver function should be monitored.
- **Side Effects:** Hepatotoxicity, pulmonary toxicity, and bone marrow suppression are potential methotrexate-related complications.

Tips & Pearls:
- Methotrexate is a cornerstone of rheumatoid arthritis treatment but requires careful monitoring of liver function and blood counts.
- Folic acid reduces methotrexate toxicity without affecting its efficacy.
- Patients should be educated to take methotrexate weekly, not daily.

Pitfalls to Avoid:

- Misinterpreting fatigue and mouth sores as a disease flare instead of drug toxicity.
- Not prescribing or adjusting folic acid supplementation.

CASE 16: HYDROXYCHLOROQUINE IN SYSTEMIC LUPUS ERYTHEMATOSUS (SLE)

Clinical Scenario:

A 30-year-old woman with SLE has been stable on hydroxychloroquine for the past year. She presents for her routine checkup with no new complaints.

She is scheduled for her annual ophthalmologic exam.

1. What is the main long-term complication of hydroxychloroquine therapy?
   A. Renal toxicity
   B. Pulmonary fibrosis
   C. Retinal toxicity
   D. Hepatotoxicity
2. How often should patients on long-term hydroxychloroquine have ophthalmologic exams?
   A. Every 6 months

B. Every year
C. Every 2 years
D. Every 5 years

3. Which of the following is a common early symptom of hydroxychloroquine-induced retinopathy?
A. Blurry vision
B. Red-green color blindness
C. Scotomas (blind spots)
D. Night blindness

Answers:

1. **C. Retinal toxicity**
2. **B. Every year**
3. **C. Scotomas (blind spots)**

Explanation:

- **Long-term Complication:** Retinal toxicity is the most significant long-term risk of hydroxychloroquine, potentially leading to irreversible vision loss.
- **Screening:** Annual eye exams are recommended after five years of treatment or sooner if risk factors are present.
- **Early Symptoms:** Scotomas or blind spots are an early sign of retinal toxicity, warranting discontinuation of the drug.

Tips & Pearls:

- Hydroxychloroquine is generally well-tolerated, with rare side effects, but retinal toxicity can be irreversible.
- Baseline and annual eye exams are important for early detection of retinopathy.
- Hydroxychloroquine is preferred in SLE for its efficacy in preventing flares and its relatively low side effect profile.

Pitfalls to Avoid:
- Delaying or missing annual eye exams for patients on long-term hydroxychloroquine therapy.
- Not recognizing early signs of retinal toxicity, leading to vision loss.

CASE 17: LEFLUNOMIDE IN PSORIATIC ARTHRITIS

Clinical Scenario:
A 55-year-old man with psoriatic arthritis is prescribed leflunomide after methotrexate fails to adequately control his symptoms.

Three months into treatment, he reports diarrhea, weight loss, and hair thinning. His liver function tests are mildly elevated.

1. What is the most likely cause of this patient's symptoms?
   A. Psoriatic arthritis flare
   B. Leflunomide toxicity
   C. NSAID side effects
   D. Dietary changes

2. What is the most appropriate next step in managing this patient?
   A. Discontinue leflunomide
   B. Reduce the dose of leflunomide
   C. Add corticosteroids
   D. Add methotrexate

3. What is the mechanism of action of leflunomide?
   A. TNF-α inhibitor
   B. Inhibits pyrimidine synthesis

C. Inhibits folic acid metabolism
D. JAK inhibitor

Answers:
1. **B. Leflunomide toxicity**
2. **A. Discontinue leflunomide**
3. **B. Inhibits pyrimidine synthesis**

Explanation:
- **Diagnosis:** Leflunomide toxicity can manifest as diarrhea, weight loss, and liver enzyme abnormalities.
- **Management:** Discontinuation is necessary if significant toxicity occurs, especially liver enzyme elevation.
- **Mechanism:** Leflunomide works by inhibiting pyrimidine synthesis, reducing the proliferation of lymphocytes.

Tips & Pearls:
- Leflunomide is an effective alternative to methotrexate but can cause gastrointestinal symptoms and hepatotoxicity.
- Cholestyramine can be used to rapidly eliminate leflunomide in cases of severe toxicity.
- Routine monitoring of liver function tests is necessary during treatment.

Pitfalls to Avoid:
- Continuing leflunomide in the presence of significant liver enzyme elevation.
- Overlooking GI symptoms and weight loss as signs of toxicity.

CASE 18: TUMOR NECROSIS FACTOR (TNF) INHIBITORS IN ANKYLOSING SPONDYLITIS

Clinical Scenario:

A 32-year-old man with ankylosing spondylitis is started on adalimumab, a TNF inhibitor, after failing to respond adequately to NSAIDs.

Two months into therapy, he develops a cough and fever. A chest X-ray reveals diffuse bilateral infiltrates.

1. What is the most likely cause of this patient's symptoms?
   A. Pneumonia
   B. Tuberculosis reactivation
   C. Drug-induced pneumonitis
   D. Acute respiratory distress syndrome
2. What is the most appropriate next step in this patient's management?
   A. Continue adalimumab and treat with antibiotics
   B. Stop adalimumab and test for tuberculosis

C. Switch to another TNF inhibitor
D. Start corticosteroids

3. What screening test should be performed before initiating TNF inhibitors?
   A. Hepatitis B serology
   B. Tuberculin skin test or IGRA
   C. Chest X-ray
   D. Complete blood count

Answers:
1. **B. Tuberculosis reactivation**
2. **B. Stop adalimumab and test for tuberculosis**
3. **B. Tuberculin skin test or IGRA**

Explanation:
- **Diagnosis:** TNF inhibitors increase the risk of reactivating latent tuberculosis, particularly in patients who were not properly screened before therapy.
- **Management:** Stopping the TNF inhibitor and testing for tuberculosis is the next step. If positive, treatment for latent TB should be initiated before restarting therapy.
- **Screening:** Screening for latent TB with a tuberculin skin test or IGRA is mandatory before starting TNF inhibitors.

Tips & Pearls:
- TNF inhibitors are highly effective for ankylosing spondylitis but carry a risk of serious infections, including TB reactivation.
- All patients should be screened for TB before starting TNF inhibitors.
- Reactivation of TB can present with atypical symptoms, including fever, cough, and nonspecific infiltrates on chest X-ray.

Pitfalls to Avoid:
- Failing to screen for TB prior to starting TNF inhibitors.
- Not recognizing symptoms of TB reactivation in patients on immunosuppressive therapy.

CASE 19: RHEUMATOID ARTHRITIS PROGNOSIS

Clinical Scenario:

A 50-year-old woman diagnosed with rheumatoid arthritis two years ago presents for a follow-up visit. She has been on methotrexate and has achieved moderate improvement in her symptoms.

However, she reports persistent morning stiffness and joint swelling in her hands. Her ESR is 40 mm/hr, and her disease activity score indicates moderate disease activity.

1. What is the most appropriate long-term management strategy for this patient?
   A. Continue methotrexate and monitor
   B. Increase the dose of methotrexate
   C. Add a biologic agent
   D. Switch to corticosteroids

2. What factor is associated with a poorer prognosis in rheumatoid arthritis?
   A. Early treatment initiation
   B. Seropositivity for rheumatoid factor (RF)
   C. Younger age at diagnosis
   D. Low disease activity score

3. What is a common follow-up recommendation for patients on long-term methotrexate therapy?
   A. Annual eye exam
   B. Regular liver function tests
   C. Routine echocardiograms
   D. Bone density scans every year

Answers:
1. **C. Add a biologic agent**
2. **B. Seropositivity for rheumatoid factor (RF)**
3. **B. Regular liver function tests**

Explanation:

- **Management:** Given the moderate disease activity, adding a biologic agent may be warranted to control her symptoms and prevent joint damage.
- **Prognosis:** Seropositivity for RF is associated with more severe disease and worse outcomes in rheumatoid arthritis.
- **Follow-Up:** Regular monitoring of liver function tests is crucial for patients on methotrexate to detect hepatotoxicity early.

Tips & Pearls:

- Early and aggressive treatment in rheumatoid arthritis can significantly improve long-term outcomes.
- Patients should be educated about the importance of adhering to follow-up appointments and monitoring tests.
- Encourage lifestyle modifications such as exercise and weight management to improve function and quality of life.

Pitfalls to Avoid:

- Delaying the initiation of biologic therapy in patients with moderate to severe disease activity.
- Failing to monitor liver function, which can lead to unrecognized toxicity.

CASE 20: SYSTEMIC LUPUS ERYTHEMATOSUS (SLE) FOLLOW-UP

Clinical Scenario:

A 28-year-old woman with SLE has been on hydroxychloroquine and low-dose corticosteroids for the past year. She presents for a routine follow-up, reporting a recent rash and increased fatigue.

She denies joint pain but admits to increased sun exposure. Her laboratory tests show an elevated anti-dsDNA antibody level and a normal complete blood count.

1. What is the most likely explanation for this patient's increased symptoms?
   A. Medication noncompliance
   B. Disease flare due to sun exposure
   C. Infection
   D. Secondary autoimmune disorder

2. What is the most appropriate next step in management?
   A. Increase the corticosteroid dose
   B. Switch to a different DMARD
   C. Continue current therapy and schedule follow-up in 3 months

D. Start immunosuppressive therapy
3. Which of the following is an important long-term follow-up consideration for patients with SLE?
    A. Routine vaccination
    B. Annual chest X-ray
    C. Regular renal function tests
    D. Annual colonoscopy

Answers:
1. **B. Disease flare due to sun exposure**
2. **A. Increase the corticosteroid dose**
3. **C. Regular renal function tests**

Explanation:
- **Management:** Increased symptoms suggest a disease flare, likely triggered by sun exposure. Increasing corticosteroid therapy can help manage this flare.
- **Follow-Up:** Patients with SLE require regular monitoring of renal function to detect lupus nephritis early, which is a common and serious complication.
- **Education:** Patients should be educated about the importance of sun protection to prevent flares.

Tips & Pearls:
- Monitor anti-dsDNA antibody levels as they correlate with disease activity in SLE.
- Patients should be encouraged to maintain regular follow-ups even during periods of remission.
- Reinforce the importance of medication adherence and regular monitoring for potential complications.

Pitfalls to Avoid:
- Misinterpreting symptoms as solely medication side effects instead of a disease flare.
- Failing to monitor renal function, which can lead to

unrecognized renal involvement.

CASE 21: ANKYLOSING SPONDYLITIS PROGNOSIS

Clinical Scenario:

A 40-year-old male with a 5-year history of ankylosing spondylitis presents for a follow-up visit.

He reports moderate relief of symptoms with NSAIDs but has developed progressive spinal stiffness and difficulty with daily activities. His physical examination reveals limited lumbar mobility.

1. What is the most likely implication of his increasing spinal stiffness?
    A. Improved prognosis
    B. Increased risk of fractures
    C. Development of spinal deformity
    D. Requirement for surgery
2. What is the most appropriate next step in management?
    A. Continue NSAIDs
    B. Refer to physical therapy
    C. Start a TNF inhibitor
    D. Add methotrexate

3. What is a common long-term complication of ankylosing spondylitis?
   A. Osteoporosis
   B. Osteomyelitis
   C. Psoriasis
   D. Peripheral neuropathy

Answers:
1. **C. Development of spinal deformity**
2. **C. Start a TNF inhibitor**
3. **A. Osteoporosis**

Explanation:
- **Implication:** Increasing spinal stiffness in ankylosing spondylitis is associated with a poorer prognosis and potential for spinal deformity.
- **Management:** Starting a TNF inhibitor can significantly improve symptoms and function in patients with inadequate response to NSAIDs.
- **Complications:** Patients with ankylosing spondylitis are at increased risk for osteoporosis due to chronic inflammation and decreased mobility.

Tips & Pearls:
- Regular assessment of spinal mobility and function is essential for managing ankylosing spondylitis.
- Encourage patients to maintain an active lifestyle and participate in physical therapy.
- Educate patients about the importance of monitoring bone density, especially if they are on long-term corticosteroids.

Pitfalls to Avoid:

- Delaying the initiation of biologic therapy in patients with progressive disease.
- Not addressing lifestyle factors that can contribute to stiffness and decreased mobility.

CASE 22: GOUT FOLLOW-UP

Clinical Scenario:

A 60-year-old man with a history of gout is on allopurinol and colchicine for management. He presents for a follow-up visit and reports having had no gout flares in the last six months.

However, he expresses concern about recent episodes of abdominal pain and diarrhea. His uric acid level is well-controlled.

1. What is the most likely cause of this patient's gastrointestinal symptoms?
   A. Gout flare
   B. Allopurinol side effects
   C. Colchicine toxicity
   D. Dietary indiscretion

2. What is the most appropriate management step for his gastrointestinal symptoms?
   A. Continue current medications
   B. Discontinue allopurinol
   C. Reduce the dose of colchicine
   D. Start an antiemetic

3. What should be monitored during long-term therapy with allopurinol?
   A. Liver function tests
   B. Renal function tests

    C. Complete blood count
    D. Serum electrolytes

Answers:
1. **C. Colchicine toxicity**
2. **C. Reduce the dose of colchicine**
3. **B. Renal function tests**

Explanation:
- **Symptoms:** The patient's abdominal pain and diarrhea are likely due to colchicine toxicity, especially if he has not been adhering to dosing recommendations.
- **Management:** Reducing the dose of colchicine can help alleviate gastrointestinal side effects.
- **Monitoring:** Renal function should be regularly monitored in patients taking allopurinol, as it can accumulate in cases of renal impairment.

Tips & Pearls:
- Patients should be educated on the proper use and dosing of colchicine to minimize gastrointestinal side effects.
- Allopurinol is effective for long-term management of gout, but close monitoring of renal function is essential.
- Encourage patients to maintain a healthy diet low in purines to help manage uric acid levels.

Pitfalls to Avoid:
- Overlooking the signs of colchicine toxicity in patients who have gastrointestinal symptoms.
- Failing to monitor renal function, especially in older patients or those with pre-existing kidney issues.

CASE 23: DIAGNOSING RHEUMATOID ARTHRITIS(2)

Clinical Scenario:

A 45-year-old woman presents with symmetric joint pain and morning stiffness lasting over an hour.

Laboratory tests reveal a positive rheumatoid factor (RF) and elevated anti-citrullinated peptide antibodies (anti-CCP). X-rays show erosions in the hands.

1. Which laboratory finding is most specific for rheumatoid arthritis?
   A. Elevated ESR
   B. Positive RF
   C. Positive anti-CCP
   D. Low hemoglobin

2. What is the most appropriate initial imaging study for assessing joint damage in rheumatoid arthritis?
   A. MRI
   B. Ultrasound
   C. X-ray
   D. CT scan

3. What is the significance of detecting anti-CCP antibodies?
   A. Indicates severe disease
   B. Associated with a higher likelihood of erosive

disease
C. Suggests a better prognosis
D. Confirms diagnosis

Answers:
1. **C. Positive anti-CCP**
2. **C. X-ray**
3. **B. Associated with a higher likelihood of erosive disease**

Explanation:
- **Findings:** Anti-CCP is more specific for rheumatoid arthritis compared to RF and is associated with more aggressive disease.
- **Imaging:** X-rays are typically the first-line imaging modality to assess for erosive changes in the joints.
- **Prognosis:** The presence of anti-CCP antibodies suggests a higher risk of developing erosive joint damage.

Tips & Pearls:
- Early detection and treatment can significantly improve outcomes in rheumatoid arthritis.
- Consider ultrasound for assessing synovitis in patients with inconclusive findings.

Pitfalls to Avoid:
- Relying solely on RF for diagnosis; a negative RF does not rule out rheumatoid arthritis.

CASE 24: EVALUATING SYSTEMIC LUPUS ERYTHEMATOSUS (SLE)

Clinical Scenario:

A 30-year-old woman presents with fatigue, joint pain, and a facial rash. Laboratory tests show a positive antinuclear antibody (ANA) and elevated anti-double-stranded DNA (anti-dsDNA) levels.

1. What does a positive ANA indicate?
   A. Specific for SLE
   B. Non-specific autoimmune activity
   C. Requires further specific testing
   D. Confirms diagnosis of lupus

2. What is the significance of elevated anti-dsDNA levels?
   A. Indicates systemic involvement
   B. Associated with active disease and renal involvement
   C. Predicts poor prognosis
   D. Confirms the diagnosis of SLE

3. Which additional test is helpful in assessing renal involvement in SLE?

A. Chest X-ray
B. Urinalysis
C. Echocardiogram
D. MRI

Answers:

1. **B. Non-specific autoimmune activity**
2. **B. Associated with active disease and renal involvement**
3. **B. Urinalysis**

Explanation:

- **ANA:** While a positive ANA is common in SLE, it is non-specific and can be seen in various conditions.
- **Anti-dsDNA:** Elevated levels correlate with disease activity and can indicate lupus nephritis.
- **Renal Involvement:** Urinalysis can reveal proteinuria or hematuria, suggesting renal complications in SLE.

Tips & Pearls:

- Regular monitoring of anti-dsDNA levels can help assess disease activity in SLE.
- Educate patients on recognizing symptoms of flares to seek timely care.

Pitfalls to Avoid:

- Misinterpreting a positive ANA as definitive for SLE without considering clinical context.

CASE 25: INVESTIGATING GOUT

Clinical Scenario:

A 55-year-old man presents with acute podagra (big toe pain). Synovial fluid analysis shows needle-shaped crystals under polarized light microscopy.

1. What does the presence of needle-shaped crystals indicate?
   A. Calcium pyrophosphate dihydrate (CPPD) crystals
   B. Uric acid crystals
   C. Infection
   D. Rheumatoid arthritis

2. What is the most appropriate test to confirm hyperuricemia?
   A. Serum uric acid level
   B. 24-hour urine uric acid
   C. Joint aspiration
   D. X-ray

3. What lifestyle modification can help manage gout?
   A. Increase red meat consumption
   B. Reduce alcohol intake
   C. Increase fructose intake
   D. Avoid hydration

Answers:

1. **B. Uric acid crystals**
2. **A. Serum uric acid level**
3. **B. Reduce alcohol intake**

Explanation:
- **Crystals:** Needle-shaped crystals are characteristic of monosodium urate crystals seen in gout.
- **Diagnosis:** Measuring serum uric acid is crucial for diagnosing hyperuricemia.
- **Lifestyle:** Reducing alcohol intake can help lower uric acid levels and prevent flares.

Tips & Pearls:
- Early intervention with NSAIDs or colchicine can help manage acute gout attacks.
- Patient education on dietary choices is essential for long-term management.

Pitfalls to Avoid:
- Assuming high serum uric acid levels always correlate with gout attacks.

CASE 26: INVESTIGATING PSORIATIC ARTHRITIS

Clinical Scenario:
A 40-year-old man with psoriasis presents with joint pain and swelling in his fingers. Physical examination reveals dactylitis. Laboratory tests show a negative rheumatoid factor.

1. What is the most characteristic radiographic finding in psoriatic arthritis?
    A. Erosions
    B. "Pencil-in-cup" deformity
    C. Joint space narrowing
    D. Subchondral sclerosis

2. What is the role of MRI in this case?
    A. Confirm the diagnosis
    B. Assess for sacroiliitis
    C. Evaluate for bone marrow edema
    D. Both B and C

3. Which serological marker is often associated with psoriatic arthritis?
    A. Anti-CCP
    B. HLA-B27
    C. RF
    D. Anti-dsDNA

Answers:
1. **B. "Pencil-in-cup" deformity**
2. **D. Both B and C**
3. **B. HLA-B27**

Explanation:
- **Findings:** The "pencil-in-cup" deformity is a classic radiographic feature of psoriatic arthritis.
- **MRI:** Useful for detecting sacroiliitis and bone marrow edema, which can assist in diagnosing axial involvement.
- **Markers:** HLA-B27 positivity is associated with an increased risk of developing spondyloarthritis, including psoriatic arthritis.

Tips & Pearls:
- Early recognition of psoriatic arthritis can help prevent joint damage.
- Encourage patients to maintain regular follow-ups to monitor disease progression.

Pitfalls to Avoid:
- Misdiagnosing psoriatic arthritis as rheumatoid arthritis based on joint symptoms alone.

CASE 27: EVALUATING ANKYLOSING SPONDYLITIS

Clinical Scenario:
A 30-year-old male presents with chronic low back pain and stiffness, particularly worse in the morning. He reports improvement with physical activity. MRI reveals sacroiliitis.

1. What is the most useful laboratory test for assessing spondyloarthritis?
   A. Serum uric acid
   B. HLA-B27 antigen
   C. C-reactive protein
   D. Complete blood count

2. What is the primary goal of follow-up in ankylosing spondylitis?
   A. Monitor kidney function
   B. Assess response to treatment and functional status
   C. Screen for malignancy
   D. Monitor liver function

3. What is an important lifestyle recommendation for patients with ankylosing spondylitis?
   A. Avoid physical activity
   B. Engage in regular exercises and stretching
   C. Increase bed rest

    D. Limit hydration

Answers:
1. **B. HLA-B27 antigen**
2. **B. Assess response to treatment and functional status**
3. **B. Engage in regular exercises and stretching**

Explanation:
- **Testing:** HLA-B27 antigen testing helps identify individuals at risk for spondyloarthritis.
- **Follow-Up:** Monitoring functional status and treatment response is essential for managing ankylosing spondylitis.
- **Lifestyle:** Regular exercises help maintain mobility and improve quality of life.

Tips & Pearls:
- Encourage participation in physical therapy and exercise programs tailored for ankylosing spondylitis.
- Educate patients about the importance of early intervention to reduce disease progression.

Pitfalls to Avoid:
- Failing to recognize the importance of physical activity in managing symptoms.

CASE 28: INVESTIGATING SJÖGREN'S SYNDROME

Clinical Scenario:

A 50-year-old woman presents with dry eyes and dry mouth. Schirmer's test confirms reduced tear production. Laboratory tests show positive ANA and anti-Ro/SSA antibodies.

1. What is the most significant lab finding for confirming Sjögren's syndrome?
   A. Positive ANA
   B. Positive anti-Ro/SSA antibodies
   C. Positive anti-La/SSB antibodies
   D. Elevated ESR

2. Which additional test can help assess salivary gland function?
   A. Salivary gland ultrasound
   B. Lip biopsy
   C. Sialography
   D. CT scan

3. What is a potential complication of Sjögren's syndrome?
   A. Osteoporosis

B. Increased risk of lymphoma
C. Cardiovascular disease
D. Chronic kidney disease

Answers:
1. **B. Positive anti-Ro/SSA antibodies**
2. **B. Lip biopsy**
3. **B. Increased risk of lymphoma**

Explanation:
- **Findings:** Positive anti-Ro/SSA antibodies are commonly associated with Sjögren's syndrome and indicate a higher risk for complications.
- **Testing:** A lip biopsy can reveal lymphocytic infiltration of the salivary glands, supporting the diagnosis.
- **Complications:** Patients with Sjögren's syndrome are at increased risk for developing non-Hodgkin lymphoma.

Tips & Pearls:
- Educate patients about managing dry eyes and dry mouth with appropriate therapies.
- Regular monitoring for complications, including lymphoma, is crucial.

Pitfalls to Avoid:
- Failing to consider the risk of lymphoma in patients with long-standing Sjögren's syndrome.

CASE 29: INVESTIGATING OSTEOARTHRITIS

Clinical Scenario:
A 65-year-old woman presents with chronic knee pain that worsens with activity. X-rays reveal joint space narrowing and osteophytes.

1. What is the hallmark radiographic feature of osteoarthritis?
   A. Erosions
   B. Joint space narrowing
   C. Subchondral sclerosis
   D. All of the above
2. Which laboratory test is most useful in ruling out inflammatory arthritis in this patient?
   A. RF
   B. ESR
   C. CRP
   D. Complete blood count
3. What is the most appropriate initial treatment for this patient's osteoarthritis?
   A. Corticosteroids
   B. Joint aspiration
   C. NSAIDs

D. Disease-modifying antirheumatic drugs (DMARDs)

Answers:
1. **B. Joint space narrowing**
2. **A. RF**
3. **C. NSAIDs**

Explanation:
- **Radiographic Features:** Joint space narrowing and osteophytes are characteristic of osteoarthritis.
- **Testing:** RF can help differentiate between osteoarthritis and inflammatory arthritis.
- **Management:** NSAIDs are the first-line treatment for managing pain and inflammation in osteoarthritis.

Tips & Pearls:
- Encourage weight management and physical therapy to improve function and reduce symptoms.
- Regular follow-up is important to monitor disease progression and adjust treatment as needed.

Pitfalls to Avoid:
- Overlooking non-pharmacologic approaches, such as exercise and weight loss, in managing osteoarthritis.

CASE 30: INVESTIGATING DERMATOMYOSITIS

Clinical Scenario:

A 40-year-old woman presents with a rash on her eyelids and proximal muscle weakness. Laboratory tests reveal elevated muscle enzymes (CK, aldolase) and a positive anti-Jo-1 antibody.

1. What is the significance of elevated muscle enzymes in this patient?
   A. Indicates liver damage
   B. Suggests muscle inflammation
   C. Confirms dermatomyositis
   D. Indicates renal impairment

2. What is the most useful imaging study to assess muscle involvement in dermatomyositis?
   A. MRI
   B. CT scan
   C. Ultrasound
   D. X-ray

3. Which additional test can help confirm the diagnosis of dermatomyositis?
   A. Skin biopsy
   B. Muscle biopsy
   C. EMG
   D. All of the above

Answers:
1. **B. Suggests muscle inflammation**
2. **A. MRI**
3. **D. All of the above**

Explanation:
- **Muscle Enzymes:** Elevated levels of CK and aldolase indicate muscle damage or inflammation.
- **Imaging:** MRI can help identify areas of muscle edema and inflammation.
- **Confirmation:** Muscle biopsy, skin biopsy, or EMG can help confirm the diagnosis of dermatomyositis.

Tips & Pearls:
- Early diagnosis and treatment are crucial to prevent muscle damage.
- Regular monitoring of muscle function and enzyme levels can guide treatment adjustments.

Pitfalls to Avoid:
- Failing to consider dermatomyositis in patients with unexplained muscle weakness and skin rash.

CASE 31: INVESTIGATING SCLERODERMA

Clinical Scenario:

A 35-year-old woman presents with skin thickening on her fingers and Raynaud's phenomenon. Laboratory tests show positive ANA with a speckled pattern and anti-Scl-70 antibodies.

1. What is the significance of the positive anti-Scl-70 antibodies?
   A. Indicates limited scleroderma
   B. Associated with diffuse scleroderma
   C. Confirms the diagnosis
   D. Suggests renal involvement

2. What is the most appropriate imaging study to assess pulmonary involvement?
   A. Chest X-ray
   B. High-resolution CT scan of the chest
   C. Echocardiogram
   D. MRI of the chest

3. Which additional test is important in evaluating gastrointestinal involvement in scleroderma?
   A. Upper GI series
   B. Colonoscopy
   C. Esophageal manometry
   D. Abdominal ultrasound

Answers:
1. **B. Associated with diffuse scleroderma**
2. **B. High-resolution CT scan of the chest**
3. **C. Esophageal manometry**

Explanation:
- **Anti-Scl-70:** This antibody is associated with diffuse scleroderma, which typically has a worse prognosis.
- **Imaging:** High-resolution CT scan is the gold standard for assessing interstitial lung disease in scleroderma.
- **GI Testing:** Esophageal manometry can evaluate esophageal motility dysfunction, common in scleroderma patients.

Tips & Pearls:
- Regular follow-up is essential to monitor for complications, including pulmonary fibrosis.
- Encourage lifestyle modifications, such as avoiding cold exposure to manage Raynaud's phenomenon.

Pitfalls to Avoid:
- Underestimating the importance of early detection and monitoring of organ involvement in scleroderma.

CASE 32: INVESTIGATING MIXED CONNECTIVE TISSUE DISEASE (MCTD)

Clinical Scenario:

A 28-year-old woman presents with arthritis, myositis, and Raynaud's phenomenon. Laboratory tests show a positive ANA, with anti-U1 RNP antibodies.

1. What does a positive anti-U1 RNP antibody test suggest?
   A. Indicates systemic lupus erythematosus
   B. Associated with mixed connective tissue disease
   C. Confirms the diagnosis of scleroderma
   D. Indicates rheumatoid arthritis

2. Which additional test can help assess for pulmonary involvement in MCTD?
   A. Echocardiogram
   B. Pulmonary function tests
   C. Chest X-ray
   D. Sputum culture

3. What is a common complication of mixed connective tissue disease?

A. Pulmonary hypertension
B. Myocardial infarction
C. Chronic kidney disease
D. Osteoporosis

Answers:
1. **B. Associated with mixed connective tissue disease**
2. **B. Pulmonary function tests**
3. **A. Pulmonary hypertension**

Explanation:
- **Antibodies:** Positive anti-U1 RNP antibodies are characteristic of MCTD and indicate a mixed pattern of autoimmune features.
- **Testing:** Pulmonary function tests are essential for assessing lung involvement, as MCTD can lead to pulmonary complications.
- **Complications:** Patients with MCTD are at increased risk for pulmonary hypertension due to vascular involvement.

Tips & Pearls:
- Monitor symptoms regularly and adjust treatment as needed to manage overlapping features of MCTD.
- Educate patients about recognizing signs of pulmonary complications.

Pitfalls to Avoid:
- Confusing MCTD with other connective tissue diseases due to overlapping symptoms.

CASE 33: LIMITED SYSTEMIC SCLEROSIS

Clinical Scenario:

A 50-year-old woman presents with gradual onset of skin changes, primarily involving her fingers and forearms. She also reports digital ulcers and Raynaud's phenomenon. Her medical history includes intermittent joint pain but no significant organ involvement.

1. What is the characteristic feature of limited systemic sclerosis?
   A. Rapid skin thickening
   B. Skin involvement limited to the distal extremities
   C. Lung and kidney involvement
   D. Myositis

2. Which antibody is most commonly associated with limited systemic sclerosis?
   A. Anti-Scl-70
   B. Anti-Ro/SSA
   C. Anti-centromere
   D. Anti-U1 RNP

3. What is the primary concern regarding the management of this patient's digital ulcers?
   A. Infection
   B. Gangrene
   C. Pain management
   D. Need for surgical intervention

Answers:

1. **B. Skin involvement limited to the distal extremities**
2. **C. Anti-centromere**
3. **A. Infection**

Explanation:
- **Findings:** In limited systemic sclerosis, skin involvement typically starts distally and progresses slowly, often with minimal internal organ involvement.
- **Antibodies:** Anti-centromere antibodies are commonly found in patients with limited disease.
- **Management:** Digital ulcers can lead to infections, requiring prompt care to prevent complications.

Tips & Pearls:
- Encourage patients to avoid cold exposure to manage Raynaud's phenomenon effectively.
- Regular monitoring of skin changes and digital ulcers is essential for preventing complications.

Pitfalls to Avoid:
- Underestimating the risk of infection in patients with digital ulcers.

CASE 34: LARGE VESSEL VASCULITIS

Clinical Scenario:

A 70-year-old man presents with a new headache, jaw claudication, and vision changes. He reports fatigue and unexplained weight loss. Temporal artery biopsy shows giant cell arteritis.

1. What is the primary concern associated with giant cell arteritis?
   A. Pulmonary embolism
   B. Permanent vision loss
   C. Renal failure
   D. Cardiomyopathy

2. What is the first-line treatment for giant cell arteritis?
   A. Aspirin
   B. Corticosteroids
   C. Methotrexate
   D. Anticoagulation

3. Which of the following is a common complication of untreated giant cell arteritis?
   A. Stroke
   B. Myocardial infarction
   C. Aortic dissection
   D. Visual impairment

Answers:

1. **B. Permanent vision loss**
2. **B. Corticosteroids**
3. **D. Visual impairment**

Explanation:
- **Complications:** Giant cell arteritis can lead to irreversible vision loss if not treated promptly.
- **Management:** Corticosteroids are the cornerstone of treatment to reduce inflammation and prevent complications.

Tips & Pearls:
- Urgent initiation of corticosteroids is crucial to prevent vision loss in suspected cases.
- Regular follow-up is necessary to monitor symptoms and adjust therapy.

Pitfalls to Avoid:
- Delaying treatment based on incomplete diagnostic criteria can lead to serious complications.

CASE 35: DIFFUSE SYSTEMIC SCLEROSIS

Clinical Scenario:

A 40-year-old man presents with widespread skin thickening, including his trunk and proximal extremities. He reports fatigue, shortness of breath, and recent onset of dysphagia. Laboratory tests show elevated anti-Scl-70 antibodies.

1. What is a hallmark feature of diffuse systemic sclerosis?
   A. Skin changes occurring over years
   B. Early involvement of internal organs
   C. Predominantly distal skin involvement
   D. Low risk of pulmonary complications

2. Which complication is most likely to occur in this patient due to his symptoms?
   A. Pulmonary hypertension
   B. Interstitial lung disease
   C. Renal crisis
   D. All of the above

3. What is the most appropriate initial management strategy for his pulmonary symptoms?
   A. Corticosteroids
   B. Immunosuppressants
   C. Pulmonary rehabilitation
   D. Oxygen therapy

Answers:

1. **B. Early involvement of internal organs**
2. **D. All of the above**
3. **C. Pulmonary rehabilitation**

Explanation:
- **Features:** Diffuse systemic sclerosis is characterized by rapid skin changes and early internal organ involvement, including pulmonary complications.
- **Complications:** Patients are at risk for pulmonary hypertension, interstitial lung disease, and renal crisis.
- **Management:** Pulmonary rehabilitation can improve symptoms and quality of life in patients with lung involvement.

Tips & Pearls:
- Regularly assess lung function and monitor for signs of pulmonary complications.
- Encourage patients to engage in gentle physical activity as tolerated.

Pitfalls to Avoid:
- Delaying treatment for pulmonary complications due to a focus on skin symptoms.

CASE 36: REGIONAL PAIN SYNDROMES

Clinical Scenario:

A 28-year-old woman presents with chronic pain in her left arm after a minor injury. She reports swelling, changes in skin color, and hypersensitivity to touch. A diagnosis of complex regional pain syndrome (CRPS) is considered.

1. What is a key feature of complex regional pain syndrome (CRPS)?
   A. Acute inflammatory response
   B. Symmetrical pain distribution
   C. Autonomic dysfunction
   D. Complete resolution with rest

2. Which treatment is considered effective for managing CRPS?
   A. Rest and immobilization
   B. Antidepressants
   C. Physical therapy and desensitization
   D. Surgical intervention

3. What is an important aspect of patient education in CRPS?
   A. Avoiding all physical activity
   B. Understanding the chronic nature of the condition
   C. Focusing solely on medication management
   D. Ignoring pain signals

Answers:

1. **C. Autonomic dysfunction**
2. **C. Physical therapy and desensitization**
3. **B. Understanding the chronic nature of the condition**

Explanation:
- **Features:** CRPS is characterized by pain, swelling, and autonomic changes following an injury.
- **Management:** Early intervention with physical therapy is crucial to prevent disability.
- **Education:** Patients should understand that CRPS can be chronic and may require a multidisciplinary approach.

Tips & Pearls:
- Encourage gradual desensitization and movement to improve function.
- Consider a referral to a pain specialist for comprehensive management.

Pitfalls to Avoid:
- Overlooking the psychological impact of chronic pain on patients with CRPS.

CASE 37: KAWASAKI DISEASE

Clinical Scenario:

A 5-year-old boy is admitted to the hospital with a high fever lasting more than five days, conjunctival injection, and a strawberry tongue. He also has a rash and swollen cervical lymph nodes. His parents report no recent illnesses.

1. What is the hallmark symptom of Kawasaki disease?
   A. Fever
   B. Rash
   C. Conjunctivitis
   D. Lymphadenopathy

2. What is the most serious complication associated with Kawasaki disease?
   A. Myocarditis
   B. Coronary artery aneurysm
   C. Stroke
   D. Pulmonary embolism

3. What is the initial treatment for Kawasaki disease?
   A. Corticosteroids
   B. Intravenous immunoglobulin (IVIG)
   C. Aspirin
   D. Methotrexate

Answers:

1. **A. Fever**
2. **B. Coronary artery aneurysm**

3. **B. Intravenous immunoglobulin (IVIG)**

Explanation:
- **Symptoms:** Kawasaki disease is characterized by prolonged fever and mucocutaneous symptoms.
- **Complications:** The most significant risk is the development of coronary artery aneurysms.
- **Management:** IVIG is the cornerstone of treatment to reduce inflammation and prevent coronary complications.

Tips & Pearls:
- Aspirin is used in the acute phase for fever and inflammation management.
- Regular follow-up with echocardiograms is essential to monitor for cardiac complications.

Pitfalls to Avoid:
- Delaying treatment due to misdiagnosis can increase the risk of serious cardiovascular complications.

CASE 38: MANAGING COMPLICATIONS OF SYSTEMIC SCLEROSIS

Clinical Scenario:

A 55-year-old woman with a history of diffuse systemic sclerosis presents with new-onset hypertension and hematuria. She has experienced worsening fatigue and edema in her lower extremities.

1. What is the most concerning complication in this patient related to her symptoms?
   A. Renal crisis
   B. Cardiac involvement
   C. Gastrointestinal complications
   D. Pulmonary hypertension

2. What is the first-line treatment for managing renal crisis in systemic sclerosis?
   A. Calcium channel blockers
   B. ACE inhibitors
   C. Corticosteroids
   D. Dialysis

3. Which additional test should be performed to assess for renal involvement?
   A. Urinalysis
   B. Serum creatinine
   C. Kidney ultrasound

D. All of the above

Answers:
1. **A. Renal crisis**
2. **B. ACE inhibitors**
3. **D. All of the above**

Explanation:
- **Complications:** Renal crisis is a significant concern in patients with diffuse systemic sclerosis, presenting as hypertension and hematuria.
- **Management:** ACE inhibitors are the first-line treatment for controlling hypertension and preventing renal failure.
- **Testing:** Comprehensive evaluation, including urinalysis, serum creatinine, and imaging, is necessary to assess renal function and structure.

Tips & Pearls:
- Monitor blood pressure closely in patients with systemic sclerosis to detect renal complications early.
- Educate patients on the signs of renal crisis for prompt intervention.

Pitfalls to Avoid:
- Underestimating the severity of hypertension in patients with systemic sclerosis.

CASE 39: MYOFASCIAL PAIN SYNDROME

Clinical Scenario:

A 35-year-old man presents with localized muscle pain and tenderness in his right shoulder. He describes the pain as sharp and radiating down his arm. On examination, a trigger point is noted in the right trapezius muscle.

1. What is the defining feature of myofascial pain syndrome?
    A. Widespread muscle pain
    B. Trigger points in muscles
    C. Joint swelling
    D. Bone pain

2. What is the most effective treatment for myofascial pain syndrome?
    A. Corticosteroids
    B. Trigger point injections
    C. Systemic opioids
    D. Physical therapy alone

3. Which of the following is a common co-morbid condition associated with myofascial pain syndrome?
    A. Hypertension
    B. Depression
    C. Diabetes
    D. Osteoarthritis

Answers:

1. **B. Trigger points in muscles**
2. **B. Trigger point injections**
3. **B. Depression**

Explanation:
- **Features:** Myofascial pain syndrome is characterized by the presence of trigger points that refer pain to other areas.
- **Management:** Trigger point injections and physical therapy can effectively relieve pain and restore function.
- **Co-morbidities:** Depression is commonly associated with chronic pain conditions, including myofascial pain.

Tips & Pearls:
- Educate patients about the importance of posture and ergonomics to prevent recurrence.
- Encourage relaxation techniques to reduce muscle tension.

Pitfalls to Avoid:
- Misdiagnosing myofascial pain as purely joint or nerve-related pain.

CASE 40: PAGET'S DISEASE

Clinical Scenario:

A 70-year-old man presents with persistent bone pain in his pelvis and lower back. He reports that the pain has progressively worsened over the past few months. An X-ray shows abnormal bone enlargement and thickening.

1. What is the most likely diagnosis for this patient?
   A. Osteoporosis
   B. Paget's disease of bone
   C. Osteosarcoma
   D. Metastatic bone disease

2. Which of the following is a common complication of Paget's disease?
   A. Fractures
   B. Osteomyelitis
   C. Bone tumors
   D. All of the above

3. What is the first-line treatment for symptomatic Paget's disease?
   A. NSAIDs
   B. Bisphosphonates
   C. Calcitonin
   D. Corticosteroids

Answers:
1. **B. Paget's disease of bone**
2. **A. Fractures**
3. **B. Bisphosphonates**

Explanation:
- **Diagnosis:** Paget's disease is characterized by abnormal bone remodeling, leading to pain and deformities.
- **Complications:** Patients are at increased risk for fractures due to weakened bone structure.
- **Management:** Bisphosphonates are effective in reducing bone pain and preventing complications.

Tips & Pearls:
- Monitor alkaline phosphatase levels to assess treatment response.
- Encourage weight-bearing exercises to maintain bone strength.

Pitfalls to Avoid:
- Misdiagnosing Paget's disease as osteoarthritis or other conditions.

CASE 41: SOFT TISSUE RHEUMATISM

Clinical Scenario:

A 50-year-old woman presents with diffuse musculoskeletal pain, particularly in her shoulders and hips, along with morning stiffness lasting about an hour. She has no significant joint swelling, and lab tests are unremarkable.

1. What is the most likely diagnosis for this patient?
   A. Rheumatoid arthritis
   B. Fibromyalgia
   C. Osteoarthritis
   D. Polymyalgia rheumatica

2. Which of the following is a characteristic symptom of fibromyalgia?
   A. Joint swelling
   B. Specific tender points
   C. Morning stiffness lasting several hours
   D. All of the above

3. What is the first-line treatment for fibromyalgia?
   A. Opioids
   B. SSRIs
   C. Exercise therapy
   D. Corticosteroids

Answers:

1. **D. Polymyalgia rheumatica**
2. **B. Specific tender points**

3. **C. Exercise therapy**

Explanation:
- **Diagnosis:** Polymyalgia rheumatica presents with pain and stiffness, especially in the proximal muscles, with normal laboratory findings.
- **Symptoms:** Fibromyalgia is characterized by widespread pain and specific tender points, with fatigue being common.
- **Management:** Exercise and physical therapy are key components of treatment for fibromyalgia.

Tips & Pearls:
- Encourage patients to engage in regular, low-impact exercise to improve symptoms.
- Educate patients about sleep hygiene and stress management techniques.

Pitfalls to Avoid:
- Overlooking the psychological component of fibromyalgia and soft tissue rheumatism.

CASE 42: LONG-TERM MANAGEMENT OF SYSTEMIC SCLEROSIS

Clinical Scenario:

A 60-year-old man with limited systemic sclerosis has been stable for several years but now reports increasing fatigue and new-onset dyspnea with exertion. He has a history of Raynaud's phenomenon and digital ulcers but no prior lung issues.

1. What should be the first step in evaluating this patient's new symptoms?
   A. Cardiac MRI
   B. High-resolution CT scan of the chest
   C. Pulmonary function tests
   D. Echocardiogram

2. Which of the following is a common complication in patients with limited systemic sclerosis?
   A. Sclerodactyly
   B. Pulmonary fibrosis
   C. Myositis
   D. Heart failure

3. What is an important aspect of the long-term management of systemic sclerosis?
   A. Regular screening for lung involvement
   B. Immediate immunosuppressive therapy
   C. Complete avoidance of physical activity

　　　　D. Annual kidney function tests

Answers:
1. **C. Pulmonary function tests**
2. **B. Pulmonary fibrosis**
3. **A. Regular screening for lung involvement**

Explanation:
- **Evaluation:** Pulmonary function tests help assess for restrictive lung disease, a common complication in systemic sclerosis.
- **Complications:** While limited systemic sclerosis often has less severe organ involvement, pulmonary fibrosis can still occur.
- **Management:** Regular monitoring for pulmonary complications is critical for effective long-term care.

Tips & Pearls:
- Encourage patients to report any new symptoms promptly for early evaluation and management.
- Lifestyle modifications, including smoking cessation and pulmonary rehabilitation, can significantly improve outcomes.

Pitfalls to Avoid:
- Failing to consider pulmonary complications in patients with limited systemic sclerosis.

CASE 43: POLYMYOSITIS

Clinical Scenario:

A 45-year-old woman presents with progressive proximal muscle weakness over the past few months. She reports difficulty climbing stairs and lifting her arms. Laboratory tests show elevated creatine kinase (CK) levels and positive anti-Jo-1 antibodies.

1. What is the most likely diagnosis for this patient?
   A. Dermatomyositis
   B. Polymyositis
   C. Inclusion body myositis
   D. Myasthenia gravis

2. Which additional test is essential for confirming the diagnosis?
   A. MRI of the muscles
   B. Muscle biopsy
   C. Electromyography (EMG)
   D. Genetic testing

3. What is the first-line treatment for polymyositis?
   A. Methotrexate
   B. Corticosteroids
   C. Azathioprine
   D. Rituximab

Answers:

1. **B. Polymyositis**
2. **B. Muscle biopsy**
3. **B. Corticosteroids**

Explanation:

- **Diagnosis:** Polymyositis is characterized by proximal muscle weakness and elevated muscle enzymes.
- **Testing:** A muscle biopsy typically shows inflammatory infiltrates, confirming the diagnosis.
- **Management:** Corticosteroids are the initial treatment for reducing inflammation.

Tips & Pearls:

- Regular monitoring of muscle strength and CK levels helps assess treatment response.
- Consider physical therapy to maintain muscle function.

Pitfalls to Avoid:

- Failing to differentiate polymyositis from other muscle disorders, like dermatomyositis.

CASE 44: DERMATOMYOSITIS(2)

Clinical Scenario:

A 38-year-old woman presents with a heliotrope rash and muscle weakness, including difficulty swallowing. Laboratory tests show elevated CK levels and positive anti-Mi-2 antibodies.

1. What is the characteristic skin manifestation of dermatomyositis?
   A. Gottron's papules
   B. Malar rash
   C. Heliotrope rash
   D. Bullous pemphigoid

2. Which of the following is a common associated condition with dermatomyositis?
   A. Diabetes mellitus
   B. Malignancy
   C. Hypertension
   D. Hypothyroidism

3. What is the recommended treatment for dermatomyositis?
   A. Nonsteroidal anti-inflammatory drugs (NSAIDs)
   B. Methotrexate
   C. Corticosteroids
   D. Plasmapheresis

Answers:
1. **C. Heliotrope rash**
2. **B. Malignancy**
3. **C. Corticosteroids**

Explanation:
- **Skin Manifestations:** The heliotrope rash is a classic finding in dermatomyositis, often accompanied by Gottron's papules.
- **Associations:** Dermatomyositis is associated with an increased risk of malignancy, especially in adults.
- **Management:** Corticosteroids are the first-line treatment for managing muscle inflammation and skin changes.

Tips & Pearls:
- Monitor for underlying malignancies in patients with new-onset dermatomyositis.
- Referral to a dermatologist may be beneficial for skin management.

Pitfalls to Avoid:
- Overlooking potential malignancies in patients with dermatomyositis symptoms.

CASE 45: MEDIUM VESSEL VASCULITIS

Clinical Scenario:

A 45-year-old woman presents with recurrent abdominal pain, renal impairment, and a purpuric rash on her lower extremities. Laboratory tests reveal a positive ANCA test and elevated creatinine levels.

1. What condition is characterized by medium vessel vasculitis with renal involvement and abdominal pain?
   A. Takayasu arteritis
   B. Polyarteritis nodosa
   C. Wegener's granulomatosis
   D. Churg-Strauss syndrome
2. Which imaging study is most useful for assessing renal artery involvement in this patient?
   A. CT angiography
   B. MRI
   C. Ultrasound
   D. Plain X-ray
3. What is the first-line treatment for polyarteritis nodosa?
   A. High-dose corticosteroids
   B. Methotrexate
   C. Cyclophosphamide
   D. Azathioprine

Answers:

1. **B. Polyarteritis nodosa**
2. **A. CT angiography**
3. **A. High-dose corticosteroids**

Explanation:

- **Diagnosis:** Polyarteritis nodosa affects medium-sized arteries and can present with systemic symptoms, renal impairment, and skin findings.
- **Imaging:** CT angiography helps visualize renal artery involvement.
- **Management:** High-dose corticosteroids are the first-line treatment to control inflammation and prevent further organ damage.

Tips & Pearls:

- Monitor kidney function and symptoms closely to assess treatment response.
- Referral to a rheumatologist is often beneficial for ongoing management.

Pitfalls to Avoid:

- Failing to recognize the systemic nature of medium vessel vasculitis can delay treatment.

CASE 46: SMALL VESSEL VASCULITIS

Clinical Scenario:

A 30-year-old male presents with hemoptysis, hematuria, and palpable purpura on his lower extremities. Laboratory tests reveal positive c-ANCA with anti-PR3 antibodies, and a lung biopsy shows granulomatous inflammation.

1. What is the most likely diagnosis for this patient?
   A. Microscopic polyangiitis
   B. Granulomatosis with polyangiitis (Wegener's)
   C. Churg-Strauss syndrome
   D. Essential mixed cryoglobulinemia

2. What is the primary treatment for granulomatosis with polyangiitis?
   A. High-dose corticosteroids
   B. Methotrexate
   C. Cyclophosphamide
   D. Plasmapheresis

3. Which of the following is a common complication of untreated granulomatosis with polyangiitis?
   A. Heart failure
   B. Chronic kidney disease
   C. Pulmonary fibrosis
   D. All of the above

Answers:

1. **B. Granulomatosis with polyangiitis (Wegener's)**

2. **C. Cyclophosphamide**
3. **D. All of the above**

Explanation:
- **Diagnosis:** Granulomatosis with polyangiitis commonly presents with respiratory and renal involvement along with ANCA positivity.
- **Management:** Cyclophosphamide is often used for induction therapy in severe cases to control systemic inflammation.
- **Complications:** If left untreated, the condition can lead to serious complications, including kidney failure and lung damage.

Tips & Pearls:
- Early intervention is critical to prevent organ damage in patients with ANCA-associated vasculitis.
- Close monitoring of renal function and respiratory symptoms is essential during treatment.

Pitfalls to Avoid:
- Delaying diagnosis and treatment can lead to irreversible organ damage.

CASE 47: FIBROMYALGIA(2)

Clinical Scenario:

A 45-year-old woman presents with widespread pain for the past six months, along with fatigue and sleep disturbances. She notes that her symptoms worsen with stress. On examination, multiple tender points are noted.

1. Which of the following is a common trigger for fibromyalgia symptoms?
   A. Exercise
   B. Stress
   C. Healthy diet
   D. Routine sleep

2. What is the most appropriate first-line medication for managing fibromyalgia?
   A. Gabapentin
   B. Duloxetine
   C. Methotrexate
   D. Prednisone

3. What lifestyle modification can significantly help manage fibromyalgia symptoms?
   A. Sedentary lifestyle
   B. Regular aerobic exercise
   C. High-calorie diet
   D. Isolation from social activities

Answers:
1. **B. Stress**
2. **B. Duloxetine**
3. **B. Regular aerobic exercise**

Explanation:
- **Triggers:** Stress can exacerbate fibromyalgia symptoms, leading to increased pain and fatigue.
- **Management:** Duloxetine is an effective first-line treatment for fibromyalgia, addressing both pain and mood.
- **Lifestyle:** Regular exercise has been shown to improve symptoms and overall well-being.

Tips & Pearls:
- Encourage a multidisciplinary approach, including physical therapy and counseling.
- Discuss cognitive-behavioral therapy as an adjunct treatment for managing stress and pain.

Pitfalls to Avoid:
- Focusing solely on pharmacologic treatments without considering lifestyle modifications.

CASE 48: JUVENILE IDIOPATHIC ARTHRITIS (JIA)

Clinical Scenario:

A 10-year-old girl presents with persistent joint pain and swelling in her knees and wrists for the past three months. She experiences morning stiffness lasting about 30 minutes and has been increasingly fatigued. Laboratory tests show elevated inflammatory markers.

1. What is the most likely diagnosis for this patient?
   A. Reactive arthritis
   B. Juvenile idiopathic arthritis (JIA)
   C. Systemic lupus erythematosus (SLE)
   D. Osteomyelitis

2. Which subtype of JIA is characterized by fewer than five joints affected in the first six months?
   A. Polyarticular JIA
   B. Oligoarticular JIA
   C. Systemic JIA
   D. Psoriatic arthritis

3. What is the first-line treatment for managing JIA symptoms?
   A. Methotrexate
   B. Corticosteroids
   C. Nonsteroidal anti-inflammatory drugs (NSAIDs)

D. Biologic agents

Answers:
1. **B. Juvenile idiopathic arthritis (JIA)**
2. **B. Oligoarticular JIA**
3. **C. Nonsteroidal anti-inflammatory drugs (NSAIDs)**

Explanation:
- **Diagnosis:** JIA is characterized by arthritis in one or more joints lasting more than six weeks in children under 16.
- **Subtypes:** Oligoarticular JIA affects fewer than five joints, usually large joints.
- **Management:** NSAIDs are typically the first-line treatment for pain and inflammation.

Tips & Pearls:
- Regular follow-up is crucial for monitoring disease progression and treatment response.
- Encourage physical therapy to maintain joint function and mobility.

Pitfalls to Avoid:
- Failing to recognize systemic features of JIA, such as fever or rash, can delay diagnosis.

CASE 49: SYSTEMIC JUVENILE IDIOPATHIC ARTHRITIS (SJIA)

Clinical Scenario:

A 7-year-old boy is brought to the clinic with recurrent fevers, a salmon-colored rash, and swelling in multiple joints. His parents report that he appears lethargic and has lost weight over the past month. Laboratory tests reveal elevated ferritin and inflammatory markers.

1. What is the most likely diagnosis for this patient?
    A. Oligoarticular JIA
    B. Systemic juvenile idiopathic arthritis (sJIA)
    C. Infectious arthritis
    D. Henoch-Schönlein purpura

2. Which complication is particularly associated with sJIA?
    A. Osteoporosis
    B. Macrophage activation syndrome
    C. Vision loss
    D. Renal failure

3. What is the first-line treatment for sJIA?
    A. Methotrexate
    B. NSAIDs
    C. Corticosteroids
    D. Biologic therapy

Answers:
1. **B. Systemic juvenile idiopathic arthritis (sJIA)**
2. **B. Macrophage activation syndrome**
3. **C. Corticosteroids**

Explanation:
- **Diagnosis:** sJIA presents with systemic symptoms, including fever and rash, alongside arthritis.
- **Complications:** Macrophage activation syndrome is a severe complication that can arise from sJIA.
- **Management:** Corticosteroids are crucial for controlling systemic inflammation.

Tips & Pearls:
- Monitor for signs of macrophage activation syndrome in patients with sJIA.
- Coordinate care with a pediatric rheumatologist for complex cases.

Pitfalls to Avoid:
- Confusing sJIA with infections due to overlapping symptoms can lead to mismanagement.

CASE 50: OTHER PEDIATRIC RHEUMATIC CONDITIONS

Clinical Scenario:

A 12-year-old girl presents with recurrent joint pain, particularly in her knees and ankles, along with fatigue and low-grade fevers. She has a family history of autoimmune diseases. Laboratory tests show positive ANA and anti-dsDNA antibodies.

1. What condition is most likely being considered in this patient?
   A. Juvenile idiopathic arthritis
   B. Systemic lupus erythematosus (SLE)
   C. Dermatomyositis
   D. Scleroderma

2. Which of the following findings is most characteristic of systemic lupus erythematosus in children?
   A. Photosensitivity
   B. Muscle weakness
   C. Sclerodactyly
   D. Raynaud's phenomenon

3. What is the first-line treatment for mild to moderate SLE?

A. Corticosteroids
B. NSAIDs
C. Methotrexate
D. Hydroxychloroquine

Answers:
1. **B. Systemic lupus erythematosus (SLE)**
2. **A. Photosensitivity**
3. **D. Hydroxychloroquine**

Explanation:
- **Diagnosis:** SLE can present with arthritis, fatigue, and a variety of systemic symptoms in children.
- **Characteristics:** Photosensitivity is a common manifestation in pediatric SLE.
- **Management:** Hydroxychloroquine is effective for managing mild to moderate SLE and preventing flares.

Tips & Pearls:
- Educate families about the importance of sun protection and monitoring for disease flares.
- Coordinate care with a pediatric rheumatologist for comprehensive management.

Pitfalls to Avoid:
- Overlooking the possibility of SLE in children with joint symptoms can lead to delayed diagnosis and treatment.

CASE 51: PREGNANCY AND RHEUMATIC DISEASES

Clinical Scenario:

A 28-year-old woman with systemic lupus erythematosus (SLE) presents for preconception counseling. She has been in remission for the past year and is planning to conceive. She is concerned about the potential impact of her condition on pregnancy.

1. What is a major concern for women with SLE during pregnancy?
   A. Increased risk of miscarriage
   B. Higher likelihood of cesarean delivery
   C. Development of gestational diabetes
   D. All of the above

2. Which medication is generally considered safe to continue during pregnancy for women with SLE?
   A. Methotrexate
   B. Hydroxychloroquine
   C. NSAIDs
   D. Cyclophosphamide

3. What is the recommended monitoring during pregnancy for women with a history of SLE?
   A. Routine blood pressure checks only
   B. Regular ultrasounds and monitoring of fetal

    growth
    C. Monthly laboratory tests only
    D. No additional monitoring required

Answers:
1. **D. All of the above**
2. **B. Hydroxychloroquine**
3. **B. Regular ultrasounds and monitoring of fetal growth**

Explanation:
- **Concerns:** Women with SLE face increased risks, including miscarriage and complications during delivery.
- **Medications:** Hydroxychloroquine is generally safe and can help maintain remission during pregnancy.
- **Monitoring:** Close monitoring of maternal and fetal health is essential to manage any complications.

Tips & Pearls:
- Encourage patients to maintain regular prenatal care and communication with both obstetricians and rheumatologists.
- Discuss the importance of controlling disease activity prior to conception.

Pitfalls to Avoid:
- Discontinuing essential medications without consulting a healthcare provider can lead to disease flares.

CASE 52: GERIATRIC RHEUMATOLOGY CONSIDERATIONS

Clinical Scenario:

A 75-year-old woman presents with worsening joint pain in her hands and knees. She has a history of osteoarthritis and hypertension. She is concerned about her mobility and quality of life. On examination, she has Heberden's nodes and limited range of motion in her knees.

1. What is the most common rheumatic condition in the elderly?
   A. Rheumatoid arthritis
   B. Osteoarthritis
   C. Gout
   D. Systemic lupus erythematosus

2. Which medication is often preferred for managing osteoarthritis pain in elderly patients?
   A. Opioids
   B. NSAIDs
   C. Acetaminophen
   D. Corticosteroids

3. What should be considered when prescribing medications to older adults?
   A. Their ability to tolerate high doses
   B. Potential drug interactions

C. Their preference for alternative treatments
D. None of the above

Answers:
1. **B. Osteoarthritis**
2. **C. Acetaminophen**
3. **B. Potential drug interactions**

Explanation:
- **Conditions:** Osteoarthritis is the most prevalent rheumatic disease among older adults.
- **Management:** Acetaminophen is typically preferred due to its safety profile in elderly patients, compared to NSAIDs, which can increase the risk of gastrointestinal bleeding.
- **Considerations:** Older adults often take multiple medications, necessitating careful monitoring for interactions and side effects.

Tips & Pearls:
- Encourage weight management and low-impact exercise to improve joint function.
- Assess functional status and quality of life regularly to tailor management strategies.

Pitfalls to Avoid:
- Underestimating the impact of polypharmacy and potential adverse effects in older patients.

CASE 53: PREGNANCY WITH RHEUMATIC DISEASE

Clinical Scenario:

A 32-year-old woman with rheumatoid arthritis (RA) presents in her first trimester. She reports well-controlled symptoms on methotrexate, which she has been advised to discontinue. She is worried about managing her condition during pregnancy.

1. Which of the following statements about RA in pregnancy is true?
   A. RA symptoms typically worsen during pregnancy.
   B. Most women with RA have improved symptoms during pregnancy.
   C. Methotrexate is safe for use in pregnancy.
   D. Pregnant women with RA do not need any medication.

2. What is a preferred medication for managing RA during pregnancy?
   A. Methotrexate
   B. Sulfasalazine
   C. Corticosteroids
   D. NSAIDs

3. Which complication is more common in pregnant women with RA?
   A. Preeclampsia

B. Gestational diabetes
C. Anemia
D. All of the above

Answers:
1. **B. Most women with RA have improved symptoms during pregnancy.**
2. **C. Corticosteroids**
3. **D. All of the above**

Explanation:
- **RA and Pregnancy:** Many women experience an improvement in symptoms during pregnancy, but careful management is required.
- **Medications:** Corticosteroids are often used to manage flare-ups, while methotrexate is contraindicated during pregnancy.
- **Complications:** Pregnant women with RA are at increased risk for complications such as preeclampsia.

Tips & Pearls:
- Encourage a multidisciplinary approach involving obstetricians and rheumatologists.
- Discuss the importance of maintaining a healthy lifestyle, including nutrition and exercise.

Pitfalls to Avoid:
- Failing to adjust treatment plans in response to changes in disease activity during pregnancy.

CASE 54: GERIATRIC PATIENT WITH GOUT

Clinical Scenario:

A 68-year-old man with a history of gout presents with acute onset of severe pain in his right big toe. He reports that he has not been compliant with his dietary recommendations. On examination, the joint is swollen, red, and tender.

1. What is the most appropriate first-line treatment for acute gout attacks in older adults?
   A. Corticosteroids
   B. Colchicine
   C. NSAIDs
   D. Allopurinol

2. What dietary modification should be emphasized for patients with gout?
   A. Increased red meat consumption
   B. Increased dairy intake
   C. Decreased purine-rich foods
   D. Increased sugar intake

3. Which comorbidity should be monitored in older adults with gout?
   A. Hypertension
   B. Heart failure
   C. Diabetes
   D. All of the above

Answers:

1. **C. NSAIDs**
2. **C. Decreased purine-rich foods**
3. **D. All of the above**

Explanation:
- **Treatment:** NSAIDs are the first-line treatment for acute gout attacks, but caution is necessary due to potential side effects in older adults.
- **Dietary Changes:** Reducing purine intake can help manage uric acid levels.
- **Comorbidities:** Gout is often associated with other conditions such as hypertension and metabolic syndrome, necessitating regular monitoring.

Tips & Pearls:
- Educate patients on the importance of hydration and lifestyle changes to prevent future attacks.
- Consider urate-lowering therapy for patients with recurrent gout attacks.

Pitfalls to Avoid:
- Neglecting to assess and manage comorbid conditions in patients with gout.

CASE 55: SEPTIC ARTHRITIS

Clinical Scenario:

A 45-year-old man with a history of rheumatoid arthritis presents to the emergency department with acute swelling, redness, and severe pain in his left knee. He has a fever of 101°F. On examination, the joint is warm, tender, and has limited range of motion. Synovial fluid analysis shows purulent fluid.

1. What is the most likely diagnosis for this patient?
   A. Gout
   B. Pseudogout
   C. Septic arthritis
   D. Osteoarthritis

2. What is the most appropriate initial management for suspected septic arthritis?
   A. Start NSAIDs
   B. Perform arthrocentesis and send fluid for culture
   C. Administer corticosteroids
   D. Refer for orthopedic consultation only

3. What is the most common organism responsible for septic arthritis in adults?
   A. Streptococcus
   B. Staphylococcus aureus
   C. Escherichia coli
   D. Neisseria gonorrhoeae

Answers:

1. **C. Septic arthritis**
2. **B. Perform arthrocentesis and send fluid for culture**
3. **B. Staphylococcus aureus**

Explanation:
- **Diagnosis:** Septic arthritis is characterized by joint inflammation due to infection, typically presenting with acute pain and swelling.
- **Management:** Arthrocentesis is crucial for diagnosis and therapeutic relief, allowing for fluid analysis and culture.
- **Organisms:** Staphylococcus aureus is the most common pathogen in septic arthritis in adults.

Tips & Pearls:
- Always consider septic arthritis in any patient with acute joint swelling and fever, especially those with a history of rheumatic disease.
- Early intervention is key to preventing joint damage.

Pitfalls to Avoid:
- Delaying treatment while waiting for culture results can lead to worse outcomes.

CASE 56: CATASTROPHIC ANTIPHOSPHOLIPID SYNDROME

Clinical Scenario:

A 32-year-old woman with a known history of antiphospholipid syndrome presents with acute onset of shortness of breath and chest pain. She has recently experienced multiple thromboses. On examination, she has tachycardia and hypoxia. A CT pulmonary angiogram reveals multiple pulmonary emboli.

1. What is the most appropriate initial treatment for this patient?
   A. Start anticoagulation with heparin
   B. Administer corticosteroids
   C. Perform thrombectomy
   D. Initiate thrombolytic therapy

2. What laboratory test is essential for confirming the diagnosis of antiphospholipid syndrome?
   A. Complete blood count
   B. Antinuclear antibody (ANA)
   C. Lupus anticoagulant
   D. C-reactive protein (CRP)

3. Which of the following is a potential complication of catastrophic antiphospholipid syndrome?

A. Renal failure
B. Pulmonary hypertension
C. Stroke
D. All of the above

Answers:
1. **A. Start anticoagulation with heparin**
2. **C. Lupus anticoagulant**
3. **D. All of the above**

Explanation:
- **Management:** Immediate anticoagulation is critical to prevent further thromboembolic events.
- **Diagnosis:** The presence of lupus anticoagulant is key for diagnosing antiphospholipid syndrome.
- **Complications:** Catastrophic antiphospholipid syndrome can lead to multiple organ failure and requires aggressive management.

Tips & Pearls:
- Monitor closely for signs of organ dysfunction in patients with catastrophic antiphospholipid syndrome.
- Educate patients about the importance of adherence to anticoagulation therapy.

Pitfalls to Avoid:
- Mismanagement of anticoagulation can lead to either thrombotic or hemorrhagic complications.

CASE 57: ACUTE GOUT ATTACK WITH INFECTION

Clinical Scenario:

A 60-year-old man with a history of gout presents to the emergency department with severe pain and swelling in his right ankle. He has a fever and chills. On examination, the ankle is erythematous and extremely tender. Synovial fluid analysis reveals crystals and gram-positive cocci.

1. What is the most likely dual diagnosis for this patient?
   A. Gout and rheumatoid arthritis
   B. Gout and septic arthritis
   C. Gout and osteoarthritis
   D. Gout and pseudogout

2. What is the first-line treatment for managing this acute gout attack?
   A. Colchicine
   B. Oral corticosteroids
   C. NSAIDs
   D. Allopurinol

3. When managing septic arthritis in a patient with gout, what should be prioritized?
   A. Surgical intervention
   B. Initiation of allopurinol

C. Empirical antibiotics
D. Joint aspiration only

Answers:
1. **B. Gout and septic arthritis**
2. **C. NSAIDs**
3. **C. Empirical antibiotics**

Explanation:
- **Dual Diagnosis:** Patients with gout can develop septic arthritis, especially if they have a prior history of joint damage.
- **Management:** NSAIDs are typically the first-line treatment for gout flares, while antibiotics are essential for treating the infection.
- **Prioritization:** Addressing the infection promptly is crucial in septic arthritis.

Tips & Pearls:
- Always consider the possibility of infection in patients with gout experiencing acute joint pain and fever.
- Maintain a high index of suspicion for septic arthritis in patients with a history of gout.

Pitfalls to Avoid:
- Failing to initiate appropriate antibiotics while managing gout can lead to poor outcomes.

CASE 58: PULMONARY VASCULITIS EMERGENCY

Clinical Scenario:

A 50-year-old woman with a history of granulomatosis with polyangiitis presents with severe respiratory distress and hemoptysis. She is tachypneic, and oxygen saturation is low. A chest X-ray shows bilateral infiltrates.

1. What is the most urgent intervention for this patient?
   A. Initiate high-dose corticosteroids
   B. Start bronchodilators
   C. Administer oxygen therapy only
   D. Refer for lung transplant evaluation

2. Which laboratory test can help confirm the diagnosis?
   A. Chest CT scan
   B. ANCA (antineutrophil cytoplasmic antibody) test
   C. Serum creatinine
   D. Complete blood count

3. What complication should be monitored in patients with pulmonary vasculitis?
   A. Pulmonary fibrosis
   B. Chronic obstructive pulmonary disease (COPD)
   C. Pulmonary embolism

D. All of the above

Answers:
1. **A. Initiate high-dose corticosteroids**
2. **B. ANCA (antineutrophil cytoplasmic antibody) test**
3. **D. All of the above**

Explanation:
- **Management:** High-dose corticosteroids are critical for managing active pulmonary vasculitis to control inflammation.
- **Diagnosis:** ANCA testing is a useful marker for confirming granulomatosis with polyangiitis.
- **Complications:** Patients are at risk for various pulmonary complications due to vasculitis.

Tips & Pearls:
- Prompt recognition and management of pulmonary involvement in vasculitis can prevent significant morbidity.
- Collaborate with a pulmonologist for comprehensive care.

Pitfalls to Avoid:
- Delaying treatment in acute cases can result in irreversible lung damage.

CASE 59: ADULT STILL'S DISEASE

Clinical Scenario:

A 30-year-old woman presents to the emergency department with a high fever, joint pain in her wrists and knees, and a salmon-colored rash that appears intermittently. She reports fatigue and has noticed a significant weight loss over the past month. Laboratory tests show elevated inflammatory markers and a negative rheumatoid factor.

1. What is the most likely diagnosis for this patient?
    A. Rheumatoid arthritis
    B. Adult Still's disease
    C. Systemic lupus erythematosus
    D. Reactive arthritis
2. Which of the following findings is characteristic of Adult Still's disease?
    A. Morning stiffness
    B. Symmetrical joint involvement
    C. Daily fever spikes
    D. Osteophytes on X-ray
3. What is the initial treatment option for managing Adult Still's disease?
    A. Methotrexate
    B. Nonsteroidal anti-inflammatory drugs (NSAIDs)
    C. Corticosteroids
    D. Disease-modifying antirheumatic drugs (DMARDs)

Answers:
1. **B. Adult Still's disease**
2. **C. Daily fever spikes**
3. **B. Nonsteroidal anti-inflammatory drugs (NSAIDs)**

Explanation:
- **Diagnosis:** Adult Still's disease is characterized by quotidian fever, arthritis, and a distinctive rash.
- **Management:** NSAIDs are commonly used as first-line therapy to manage inflammation.

Tips & Pearls:
- Be vigilant for systemic symptoms like fever and rash in patients with joint pain, as these may indicate a systemic condition.
- Early recognition and treatment can prevent long-term complications.

Pitfalls to Avoid:
- Overlooking systemic features in patients presenting with isolated joint pain can delay diagnosis.

CASE 60: MIXED CONNECTIVE TISSUE DISEASE (MCTD)

Clinical Scenario:

A 25-year-old woman presents with Raynaud's phenomenon, polyarthritis, and skin changes resembling scleroderma. Laboratory tests reveal the presence of anti-U1 RNP antibodies. She reports episodes of fatigue and difficulty swallowing.

1. What is the most likely diagnosis for this patient?
   A. Systemic lupus erythematosus
   B. Mixed connective tissue disease
   C. Scleroderma
   D. Rheumatoid arthritis

2. Which symptom is often associated with MCTD?
   A. Avascular necrosis
   B. Pulmonary hypertension
   C. Dysphagia
   D. Morning stiffness

3. What is the best approach for managing MCTD?
   A. High-dose corticosteroids only
   B. Symptomatic treatment and monitoring
   C. Antimalarial medications only
   D. Immunosuppressive therapy only

Answers:

1. **B. Mixed connective tissue disease**

2. **C. Dysphagia**
3. **B. Symptomatic treatment and monitoring**

Explanation:

- **Diagnosis:** MCTD presents with features of several connective tissue diseases and is often associated with specific autoantibodies.
- **Management:** Treatment is tailored to symptoms and may include NSAIDs, corticosteroids, and other immunosuppressive agents.

Tips & Pearls:

- Recognize that MCTD can evolve over time, with symptoms of different connective tissue diseases becoming more prominent.
- Regular follow-up is important to monitor disease progression and treatment response.

Pitfalls to Avoid:

- Misclassifying MCTD as a single disease can lead to inappropriate treatment.

CASE 61: EOSINOPHILIC GRANULOMATOSIS WITH POLYANGIITIS (EGPA)

Clinical Scenario:

A 55-year-old man presents with asthma, nasal polyps, and a peripheral neuropathy characterized by numbness in his hands and feet. He has elevated eosinophils on a complete blood count and renal function tests reveal mild impairment. A biopsy of his skin shows eosinophilic infiltration.

1. What is the most likely diagnosis for this patient?
    A. Granulomatosis with polyangiitis
    B. Eosinophilic granulomatosis with polyangiitis
    C. Churg-Strauss syndrome
    D. Polyarteritis nodosa
2. What is the first-line treatment for EGPA?
    A. Methotrexate
    B. Corticosteroids
    C. Azathioprine
    D. Rituximab
3. Which of the following complications is most commonly associated with EGPA?

A. Renal failure
B. Pulmonary fibrosis
C. Cardiac involvement
D. All of the above

Answers:
1. **B. Eosinophilic granulomatosis with polyangiitis**
2. **B. Corticosteroids**
3. **D. All of the above**

Explanation:
- **Diagnosis:** EGPA presents with asthma, eosinophilia, and systemic vasculitis affecting multiple organs.
- **Management:** Corticosteroids are essential for controlling inflammation and managing symptoms.

Tips & Pearls:
- Be aware of the association between asthma and eosinophilia as a potential indicator of EGPA.
- Early treatment is crucial to prevent serious complications.

Pitfalls to Avoid:
- Failing to recognize the systemic nature of EGPA can delay appropriate treatment.

CASE 62: DMARDS IN RHEUMATOID ARTHRITIS

Clinical Scenario:

A 50-year-old woman with a diagnosis of rheumatoid arthritis for five years presents with persistent joint pain despite being on methotrexate. Her physician is considering adding a second disease-modifying antirheumatic drug (DMARD) to her regimen.

1. Which of the following DMARDs can be considered as an addition to methotrexate?
   A. Hydroxychloroquine
   B. Azathioprine
   C. Sulfasalazine
   D. All of the above

2. What is a common side effect of methotrexate that needs monitoring?
   A. Liver toxicity
   B. Bone marrow suppression
   C. Pulmonary toxicity
   D. All of the above

3. What is the recommended monitoring frequency for liver function tests in patients on methotrexate?
   A. Every month
   B. Every 3 months

C. Every 6 months
  D. Annually

Answers:
1. **D. All of the above**
2. **D. All of the above**
3. **B. Every 3 months**

Explanation:
- **DMARDs:** Hydroxychloroquine, azathioprine, and sulfasalazine are all options that can be used in conjunction with methotrexate.
- **Monitoring:** Regular monitoring of liver function, blood counts, and pulmonary function is essential while on DMARD therapy.

Tips & Pearls:
- Consider patient-specific factors (e.g., comorbidities, preferences) when selecting DMARDs.
- Educate patients about potential side effects and the importance of adherence to monitoring.

Pitfalls to Avoid:
- Neglecting to monitor for side effects can lead to significant complications.

CASE 63: BIOLOGICS IN PSORIATIC ARTHRITIS

Clinical Scenario:

A 38-year-old man with psoriatic arthritis presents with inadequate response to NSAIDs and methotrexate. He has extensive skin involvement and significant joint pain. The physician considers starting a biologic agent.

1. Which class of biologic agents is most effective for treating psoriatic arthritis?
   A. TNF inhibitors
   B. IL-6 inhibitors
   C. B-cell depleting agents
   D. IL-17 inhibitors

2. Which of the following is a common side effect of TNF inhibitors?
   A. Gastrointestinal bleeding
   B. Increased risk of infections
   C. Heart failure
   D. All of the above

3. Before starting a biologic agent, which screening test should be performed?
   A. Hepatitis B and C screening
   B. Tuberculosis screening
   C. Complete blood count

D. All of the above

Answers:
1. **A. TNF inhibitors**
2. **D. All of the above**
3. **D. All of the above**

Explanation:
- **Biologics:** TNF inhibitors are commonly used for psoriatic arthritis, but other classes like IL-17 inhibitors can also be effective.
- **Monitoring:** Patients should be screened for infections, particularly tuberculosis, before starting biologic therapy.

Tips & Pearls:
- Discuss the benefits and risks of biologic therapy with patients, emphasizing the importance of early intervention for better outcomes.
- Encourage vaccination and infection prevention strategies.

Pitfalls to Avoid:
- Failing to screen for latent infections can lead to severe complications when starting biologic therapy.

CASE 64: NOVEL THERAPIES IN SLE

Clinical Scenario:

A 28-year-old woman with systemic lupus erythematosus (SLE) presents with persistent fatigue and joint pain despite treatment with hydroxychloroquine and corticosteroids. The physician is considering a novel therapy.

1. Which of the following novel therapies is approved for treating SLE?
   A. Belimumab
   B. Rituximab
   C. Abatacept
   D. All of the above

2. What is the mechanism of action of belimumab?
   A. B-cell inhibition
   B. IL-6 inhibition
   C. TNF inhibition
   D. Complement inhibition

3. What should be monitored in patients starting belimumab?
   A. Liver function
   B. Blood pressure
   C. Infection risk
   D. All of the above

Answers:

1. **A. Belimumab**

2. **A. B-cell inhibition**
3. **C. Infection risk**

Explanation:
- **Novel Therapies:** Belimumab is a B-cell inhibitor specifically approved for treating SLE, while rituximab and abatacept may be used off-label.
- **Monitoring:** Patients should be monitored for signs of infection, especially with therapies that affect the immune system.

Tips & Pearls:
- Tailor therapy to individual patient profiles and treatment goals.
- Engage patients in shared decision-making regarding treatment options.

Pitfalls to Avoid:
- Not considering the patient's complete disease profile may lead to inadequate management.

CASE 65: MANAGING TREATMENT-RELATED COMPLICATIONS

Clinical Scenario:

A 60-year-old woman with osteoarthritis has been taking NSAIDs for chronic pain. She presents with new-onset abdominal pain and signs of gastrointestinal bleeding.

1. What is the most likely complication from long-term NSAID use?
   A. Hepatic failure
   B. Peptic ulcer disease
   C. Renal failure
   D. Cardiovascular events

2. What is the first step in managing this patient?
   A. Perform an endoscopy
   B. Discontinue NSAIDs
   C. Start proton pump inhibitors (PPIs)
   D. Refer for surgery

3. Which of the following medications can be used as a safer alternative for managing pain in patients with a history of gastrointestinal complications?
   A. Acetaminophen
   B. COX-2 inhibitors

C. Topical NSAIDs
D. All of the above

Answers:
1. **B. Peptic ulcer disease**
2. **B. Discontinue NSAIDs**
3. **D. All of the above**

Explanation:
- **Complications:** Long-term NSAID use can lead to gastrointestinal issues, including peptic ulcers and bleeding.
- **Management:** Discontinuation of NSAIDs and initiation of PPIs can help manage symptoms and prevent further complications.

Tips & Pearls:
- Assess patients for risk factors for gastrointestinal complications when prescribing NSAIDs.
- Consider alternative pain management strategies for patients at risk.

Pitfalls to Avoid:
- Ignoring gastrointestinal symptoms in patients on NSAIDs can lead to serious complications.

CASE 66: COLLABORATIVE CARE FOR A PATIENT WITH OSTEOARTHRITIS

Clinical Scenario:

A 65-year-old man with knee osteoarthritis presents with severe pain, limited mobility, and difficulty performing daily activities. His rheumatologist recommends a multidisciplinary approach, including referrals to orthopedics and physical therapy.

1. What is the primary goal of referring this patient to physical therapy?
   A. Pain relief through medication
   B. Improvement of joint function and mobility
   C. Surgical intervention
   D. Diagnostic imaging

2. Which of the following interventions might an orthopedic surgeon recommend for this patient?
   A. Corticosteroid injection
   B. Knee arthroscopy
   C. Total knee replacement
   D. All of the above

3. What is a key component of the interdisciplinary

care plan for this patient?
A. Education on self-management techniques
B. Sole reliance on medication
C. Avoiding exercise
D. Exclusively using heat therapy

Answers:
1. **B. Improvement of joint function and mobility**
2. **D. All of the above**
3. **A. Education on self-management techniques**

Explanation:
- **Collaboration:** An interdisciplinary approach combines the expertise of rheumatologists, orthopedic surgeons, and physical therapists to improve patient outcomes.
- **Interventions:** Various treatment options, including physical therapy and potential surgical procedures, should be discussed in the care plan.

Tips & Pearls:
- Encourage open communication among all team members to coordinate care effectively.
- Involve the patient in decision-making to enhance adherence to the treatment plan.

Pitfalls to Avoid:
- Failing to coordinate care can lead to fragmented treatment and poor patient outcomes.

CASE 67: RHEUMATOID ARTHRITIS AND ORTHOPEDIC MANAGEMENT

Clinical Scenario:

A 52-year-old woman with rheumatoid arthritis presents with significant joint deformities in her hands and feet. She is experiencing persistent pain and functional limitations. The rheumatologist decides to collaborate with an orthopedic surgeon for further management.

1. Which surgical intervention may be considered for this patient to improve function?
   A. Synovectomy
   B. Joint fusion
   C. Joint replacement
   D. All of the above

2. What role does the physical therapist play in the management of this patient?
   A. Performing surgeries
   B. Providing patient education on adaptive techniques
   C. Diagnosing conditions

D. Prescribing medications
3. What is an important factor to consider when planning surgery for patients with rheumatoid arthritis?
A. Their age only
B. The duration of disease and current disease activity
C. Previous surgeries only
D. The patient's occupation only

Answers:
1. **D. All of the above**
2. **B. Providing patient education on adaptive techniques**
3. **B. The duration of disease and current disease activity**

Explanation:
- **Interdisciplinary Role:** Collaboration between rheumatologists and orthopedic surgeons is crucial for managing complex cases of rheumatoid arthritis.
- **Surgical Options:** Various surgical interventions can improve function and alleviate pain, while physical therapy helps with rehabilitation.

Tips & Pearls:
- Ensure a comprehensive preoperative assessment to optimize surgical outcomes.
- Use a team approach to address both surgical and rehabilitative needs.

Pitfalls to Avoid:
- Not considering the patient's overall disease activity can lead to suboptimal surgical outcomes.

CASE 68: FIBROMYALGIA AND MULTIDISCIPLINARY APPROACH

Clinical Scenario:

A 40-year-old woman is diagnosed with fibromyalgia. She experiences widespread pain, fatigue, and cognitive difficulties. The rheumatologist refers her to a pain specialist, psychologist, and physical therapist for comprehensive management.

1. Which type of therapy might a psychologist recommend for managing fibromyalgia symptoms?
    A. Cognitive-behavioral therapy
    B. Physical therapy
    C. Pharmacologic therapy
    D. Occupational therapy

2. What is a common goal of physical therapy in the management of fibromyalgia?
    A. Increase pain levels
    B. Decrease activity levels
    C. Enhance physical conditioning and flexibility
    D. Focus solely on medication management

3. Which medication class is often used in managing fibromyalgia?
    A. Opioids

B. Antidepressants
   C. NSAIDs
   D. Corticosteroids

Answers:
1. **A. Cognitive-behavioral therapy**
2. **C. Enhance physical conditioning and flexibility**
3. **B. Antidepressants**

Explanation:
- **Multidisciplinary Management:** Fibromyalgia benefits from a team approach, integrating psychological support, physical therapy, and pharmacological treatments.
- **Therapeutic Goals:** Each specialty addresses different aspects of the disease, improving overall patient well-being.

Tips & Pearls:
- Educate patients about the multifaceted nature of fibromyalgia and the importance of a collaborative approach.
- Monitor the effectiveness of each intervention and adjust the treatment plan as needed.

Pitfalls to Avoid:
- Neglecting the psychological component of fibromyalgia management can hinder recovery.

CASE 69: INTERDISCIPLINARY APPROACH IN GOUT MANAGEMENT

Clinical Scenario:

A 55-year-old man with recurrent gout flares presents to his rheumatologist. Despite pharmacologic management, he continues to experience painful attacks. The rheumatologist decides to refer him to a nutritionist and an orthopedic specialist for further evaluation.

1. What dietary modification might a nutritionist suggest for managing gout?
   A. Increase intake of purine-rich foods
   B. Limit alcohol consumption
   C. Decrease fluid intake
   D. Avoid low-fat dairy products

2. What is the role of the orthopedic specialist in this patient's care?
   A. Prescribing urate-lowering therapy
   B. Evaluating for joint damage and potential surgery
   C. Conducting dietary counseling
   D. Diagnosing the condition

3. Which medication is commonly used for long-term management of gout?

A. Colchicine
B. Allopurinol
C. Indomethacin
D. Prednisone

Answers:
1. **B. Limit alcohol consumption**
2. **B. Evaluating for joint damage and potential surgery**
3. **B. Allopurinol**

Explanation:
- **Collaborative Management:** An interdisciplinary approach can address the multiple factors contributing to gout flares, including dietary habits and joint health.
- **Pharmacologic Options:** Long-term management with urate-lowering therapies is essential to prevent flares and joint damage.

Tips & Pearls:
- Encourage patients to engage in lifestyle modifications that can significantly reduce gout attacks.
- Regular follow-up with all team members is crucial for optimizing care.

Pitfalls to Avoid:
- Overlooking the importance of dietary management in gout can lead to ongoing symptoms.

CASE 70: MECHANICAL LOW BACK PAIN

Clinical Scenario:

A 45-year-old office worker presents with a 3-month history of low back pain, exacerbated by prolonged sitting and relieved by movement. She reports no radiation of pain, neurological deficits, or constitutional symptoms.

1. Which of the following is the most likely cause of this patient's low back pain?
   A. Disc herniation
   B. Muscle strain
   C. Osteoarthritis
   D. Ankylosing spondylitis

2. What initial management strategy is most appropriate for this patient?
   A. MRI of the lumbar spine
   B. Referral to a pain specialist
   C. Physical therapy and activity modification
   D. Surgical intervention

3. Which of the following is a common red flag that may indicate a more serious underlying condition?
   A. Pain worsening with movement
   B. Night pain
   C. Pain relieved by rest

       D. Localized tenderness

Answers:
1. **B. Muscle strain**
2. **C. Physical therapy and activity modification**
3. **B. Night pain**

Explanation:
- **Mechanical Pain:** This patient's symptoms are consistent with mechanical low back pain, often caused by muscle strain or ligamentous injury.
- **Management:** Initial treatment typically involves conservative measures such as physical therapy, education, and activity modification.

Tips & Pearls:
- Educate patients on the importance of maintaining activity levels while managing pain.
- Encourage ergonomic adjustments in the workplace.

Pitfalls to Avoid:
- Failing to recognize red flags can delay diagnosis and treatment of serious conditions.

CASE 71: INFLAMMATORY LOW BACK PAIN

Clinical Scenario:

A 30-year-old man presents with a 6-month history of low back pain and stiffness, particularly in the morning. He reports that the pain improves with activity but worsens after prolonged periods of rest. He has no history of injury.

1. Which condition is most likely responsible for this patient's symptoms?
   A. Mechanical strain
   B. Ankylosing spondylitis
   C. Sciatica
   D. Lumbar disc herniation
2. Which laboratory test would be most helpful in supporting a diagnosis of ankylosing spondylitis?
   A. Complete blood count (CBC)
   B. Erythrocyte sedimentation rate (ESR)
   C. HLA-B27 antigen test
   D. Creatinine kinase (CK)
3. What is the first-line treatment for this condition?
   A. Opioids
   B. NSAIDs
   C. Corticosteroids
   D. Physical therapy only

Answers:
1. **B. Ankylosing spondylitis**
2. **C. HLA-B27 antigen test**
3. **B. NSAIDs**

Explanation:
- **Inflammatory Pain:** The symptoms suggest ankylosing spondylitis, characterized by morning stiffness and improvement with activity.
- **Diagnosis:** Testing for the HLA-B27 antigen can support the diagnosis, alongside imaging studies.

Tips & Pearls:
- Early diagnosis and management of inflammatory back pain are crucial to prevent long-term complications.
- Encourage regular exercise and physical therapy to maintain mobility.

Pitfalls to Avoid:
- Delaying diagnosis of inflammatory conditions can lead to irreversible damage.

CASE 72: DIFFERENTIAL DIAGNOSIS APPROACH

Clinical Scenario:

A 50-year-old woman presents with acute low back pain following a fall. She reports shooting pain down her left leg, numbness in her foot, and difficulty walking. The pain worsens with sitting and improves with standing.

1. What is the most appropriate initial imaging study for this patient?
   A. X-ray of the lumbar spine
   B. MRI of the lumbar spine
   C. CT scan of the abdomen
   D. Ultrasound of the spine

2. Which finding would be most concerning for a herniated disc?
   A. Positive straight leg raise test
   B. Localized tenderness
   C. Pain with flexion
   D. History of previous low back pain

3. What is an important aspect of the management plan for this patient?
   A. Immediate surgical intervention

B. Use of NSAIDs and physical therapy
C. Strict bed rest
D. Avoiding all forms of exercise

Answers:
1. **B. MRI of the lumbar spine**
2. **A. Positive straight leg raise test**
3. **B. Use of NSAIDs and physical therapy**

Explanation:
- **Differential Diagnosis:** Given the acute presentation and neurological symptoms, an MRI is warranted to evaluate for a herniated disc.
- **Management:** Conservative measures including NSAIDs and physical therapy are often effective initially.

Tips & Pearls:
- Regular follow-up to assess symptom progression is important in acute low back pain cases.
- Educate the patient on the importance of staying active as tolerated.

Pitfalls to Avoid:
- Relying solely on imaging without a comprehensive clinical assessment can lead to misdiagnosis.

CASE 73: CHRONIC LOW BACK PAIN MANAGEMENT

Clinical Scenario:

A 65-year-old man with a history of chronic low back pain due to degenerative disc disease presents with a flare-up of his symptoms. He is currently on oral analgesics but is seeking more effective relief.

1. What is an appropriate next step in the management of this patient's chronic pain?
   A. Increased dosage of oral analgesics
   B. Referral for interventional pain management
   C. Immediate surgical consultation
   D. Complete cessation of all activity

2. Which of the following non-pharmacological interventions can be beneficial for chronic low back pain?
   A. Acupuncture
   B. Yoga
   C. Cognitive-behavioral therapy
   D. All of the above

3. What is a key component of a chronic pain management plan?
   A. Focus solely on medication management
   B. Emphasize multidisciplinary approaches

C. Avoid any form of physical activity
D. Rely on imaging studies to dictate treatment

Answers:
1. **B. Referral for interventional pain management**
2. **D. All of the above**
3. **B. Emphasize multidisciplinary approaches**

Explanation:
- **Chronic Management:** For chronic low back pain, a multidisciplinary approach can optimize outcomes, involving pain management specialists and physical therapists.
- **Interventions:** Various non-pharmacological interventions, including acupuncture and cognitive-behavioral therapy, can be effective.

Tips & Pearls:
- Encourage patients to set realistic goals and engage actively in their management plan.
- Regularly reassess the pain management strategy to ensure its effectiveness.

Pitfalls to Avoid:
- Relying only on pharmacological treatments without addressing lifestyle factors can lead to suboptimal results.

CASE 74: MONOARTHRITIS

Clinical Scenario:

A 28-year-old man presents with sudden onset of severe pain and swelling in his right knee. He reports no previous joint issues and denies any recent trauma. He has a fever of 101°F (38.3°C) and a notable history of gout.

1. What is the most likely diagnosis for this patient?
   A. Osteoarthritis
   B. Septic arthritis
   C. Gout
   D. Psoriatic arthritis

2. Which diagnostic test is most appropriate for confirming the diagnosis?
   A. X-ray of the knee
   B. Joint aspiration and synovial fluid analysis
   C. MRI of the knee
   D. Blood tests for rheumatoid factor

3. What immediate treatment should be initiated if septic arthritis is suspected?
   A. NSAIDs
   B. Joint injection with corticosteroids
   C. Intravenous antibiotics
   D. Physical therapy

Answers:
1. B. Septic arthritis
2. B. Joint aspiration and synovial fluid analysis
3. C. Intravenous antibiotics

Explanation:
- **Monoarthritis:** The sudden onset of knee swelling and fever suggests septic arthritis, especially in a patient with a history of gout.
- **Management:** Joint aspiration is crucial for diagnosis and treatment.

Tips & Pearls:
- Always assess for systemic symptoms in cases of monoarthritis.
- Prompt treatment of septic arthritis is essential to prevent joint damage.

Pitfalls to Avoid:
- Delaying aspiration and antibiotic treatment can lead to severe complications.

CASE 75: OLIGOARTHRITIS

Clinical Scenario:

A 32-year-old woman presents with swelling and pain in her right wrist and left knee. She reports that the symptoms started about two weeks ago and have gradually worsened. She also mentions mild fever and fatigue.

1. Which condition is most likely associated with this presentation?
   A. Rheumatoid arthritis
   B. Reactive arthritis
   C. Osteoarthritis
   D. Gout

2. What additional symptom might help narrow down the diagnosis?
   A. Morning stiffness lasting more than an hour
   B. Recent viral infection
   C. Family history of osteoarthritis
   D. Previous joint injury

3. Which investigation is essential for evaluating this patient's condition?
   A. Complete blood count (CBC)
   B. Urinalysis
   C. Joint ultrasound
   D. Antinuclear antibody (ANA) test

Answers:
1. **B. Reactive arthritis**
2. **B. Recent viral infection**
3. **A. Complete blood count (CBC)**

Explanation:
- **Oligoarthritis:** The involvement of two joints and recent symptoms suggest reactive arthritis, often triggered by an infection.
- **Workup:** A CBC can help identify any inflammatory markers.

Tips & Pearls:
- Assess for any history of recent infections, especially genitourinary or gastrointestinal.
- Encourage the patient to keep a symptom diary to track changes.

Pitfalls to Avoid:
- Overlooking the potential infectious cause can delay appropriate treatment.

CASE 76: POLYARTHRITIS

Clinical Scenario:

A 45-year-old female patient presents with symmetrical joint pain affecting her hands, wrists, and knees. She has been feeling fatigued and has lost 10 pounds over the past month without trying. On examination, she has morning stiffness lasting more than an hour.

1. What is the most likely diagnosis?
   A. Osteoarthritis
   B. Rheumatoid arthritis
   C. Systemic lupus erythematosus
   D. Fibromyalgia

2. Which laboratory test is most useful for confirming the diagnosis?
   A. Rheumatoid factor (RF)
   B. C-reactive protein (CRP)
   C. Antinuclear antibody (ANA)
   D. Erythrocyte sedimentation rate (ESR)

3. What initial treatment is recommended for this condition?
   A. Opioids
   B. Methotrexate
   C. NSAIDs
   D. Corticosteroids

Answers:
1. **B. Rheumatoid arthritis**
2. **A. Rheumatoid factor (RF)**
3. **C. NSAIDs**

Explanation:
- **Polyarthritis:** The presentation suggests rheumatoid arthritis, characterized by symmetric joint involvement and systemic symptoms.
- **Management:** NSAIDs can help manage pain and inflammation while awaiting further treatment.

Tips & Pearls:
- Educate the patient about the chronic nature of rheumatoid arthritis and the importance of early treatment.
- Regular follow-ups are essential to monitor disease activity.

Pitfalls to Avoid:
- Delaying disease-modifying therapy can lead to joint damage.

CASE 77: SYSTEMIC SYMPTOMS IN RHEUMATIC DISEASE

Clinical Scenario:

A 50-year-old man presents with persistent fatigue, low-grade fever, and unintentional weight loss over the past three months. He has joint pain in his hands and ankles that has gradually worsened. There is no history of trauma.

1. What is the most concerning differential diagnosis for this patient?
   A. Fibromyalgia
   B. Rheumatoid arthritis
   C. Malignancy
   D. Osteoarthritis

2. Which initial investigation should be performed to evaluate for systemic disease?
   A. Chest X-ray
   B. Complete blood count (CBC)
   C. Serum uric acid level
   D. Joint ultrasound

3. What additional test may help clarify the diagnosis if systemic disease is suspected?
   A. Liver function tests
   B. HLA-B27 antigen
   C. Bone marrow biopsy

D. MRI of the joints

Answers:

1. **C. Malignancy**
2. **B. Complete blood count (CBC)**
3. **D. MRI of the joints**

Explanation:

- **Systemic Symptoms:** The combination of fatigue, fever, and weight loss raises suspicion for malignancy or a serious inflammatory condition.
- **Workup:** A CBC is essential for evaluating anemia and leukocytosis, which can indicate systemic involvement.

Tips & Pearls:

- A thorough history and physical examination are crucial in identifying potential malignancies.
- Encourage the patient to report any additional symptoms that may arise.

Pitfalls to Avoid:

- Failing to consider serious underlying conditions can delay diagnosis and treatment.

ABOUT THE AUTHOR

Essam Abdelhakim

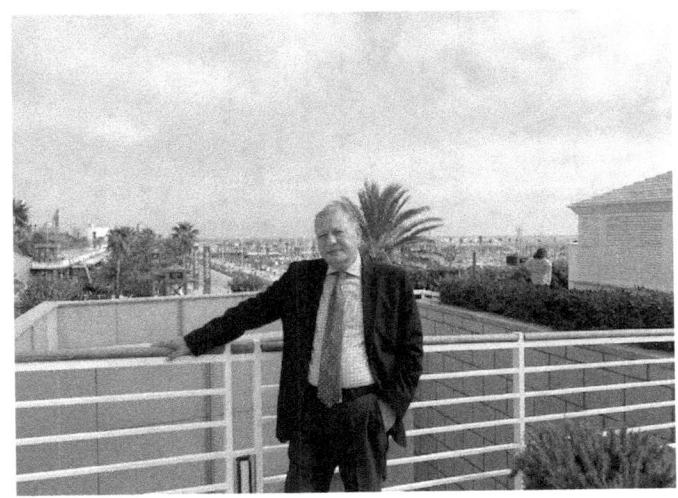

Senior Consultant and Expert in Medical Education

DISCLOSURE

Disclosure
This book has been created with the assistance of ***Artificial Intelligence (AI) tools*** and thoroughly reviewed and edited by the author to ensure clarity, relevance, and educational value.

While every effort has been made to provide accurate and up-to-date information, this content is intended solely for educational and informational purposes.
The author is a medical professional; however, the information provided in this book *is not a substitute for professional medical advice, diagnosis, or treatment.*
Readers are strongly advised to consult licensed healthcare providers or specialists for any medical concerns or conditions.

By using this book, **you acknowledge and agree** that the author shall not be held responsible or liable for any loss, damage, or harm whether physical, emotional, financial, or otherwise that may occur *as a result of the use or misuse of the information presented herein.*